OUR WORKING LIVES

A Millennium Project

by

20 Manchester Women Doctors

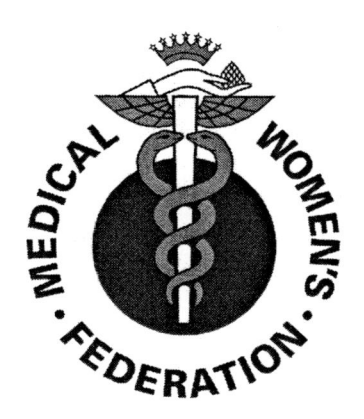

Edited by Dr Mary Hambleton

CONTENTS

	Page
Introduction	1
Acknowledgements	2
The Contributors with year of qualification and occupation:	
Dr Wray *(1932)* Pre-NHS General Practitioner	3
Dr Lempert-Barber *(1941)* Geriatrician	4
Dr Jessup *(1949)* General Practitioner	13
Dr Whale *(1955)* Microbiologist	18
Dr Roberts *(1955)* General Practitioner & Clinical Forensic Specialist	21
Miss Bannister *(1958)* Neurosurgeon	26
Miss Doig *(1962)* Paediatric Surgeon	33
Dr Anderson *(1966)* General Practitioner	37
Dr Harris *(1967)* General Practitioner	41
Professor Donnai *(1968)* Geneticist	45
Dr Lewis *(1971)* Paediatrician	54
Dr Ewing *(1978)* Paediatrician & Associate Dean, NW Region	58
Dr Ellis *(1983)* General Practitioner	64
Mrs Siddiqui *(1984)* Ophthalmologist	68
Dr Baron *(1984)* General Practitioner	70
Dr Fox *(1990)* Neurology Specialist Registrar	76
Dr Edi-Osagie *(1990)* Neonatal Paediatrics Specialist Registrar	79
Dr Blackhall *(1990)* Oncology Specialist Registrar	86
Dr Kerr-Liddell *(1999)* Paediatric Senior House Officer	91
Dr Whitehead *(2000)* Medical Senior House Officer	92
Conclusions	94
Appendix (1) – Questionnaire	99
Appendix (2) – Abbreviations	101

INTRODUCTION

The Medical Women's Federation was founded in 1917 to provide mutual support and representation for women docotors when they were still very few in number. Down the years it has become a significant force, working for reforms and developments in medical training and practice with particular reference to the needs of women doctors, who now supply a third of the medical workforce in the UK.

The Manchester branch of the Medical Women's Federation undertook to interview twenty women doctors in the Greater Manchester Area as a project for the millennium. Non-members as well as members of MWF are included.

The aim was to present an honest account of our own experiences, which we hope may be of interest to the general public and particularly to young women in the process of choosing a career. We will not try to persuade you to follow us into medicine, nor to deter you if it is truly what you want to do. We hope, however, that reading our stories will help you to determine whether medicine would be the right career for you. If you are already committed to medicine our accounts will give you some insight into possible areas of specialisation.

We have included a wide cross-section of specialties though it was not possible to represent the entire range of possible medical careers. More women doctors work in general practice than in any other field of medicine so this is reflected in the numbers. Our ages range from under thirty to over ninety.

To provide her oral history each participant was invited first to complete a short questionnaire (see Appendix 1) and then to amplify her answers whilst being recorded on tape. A transcription of the recording was sent to the participant for checking. A couple of participants replaced their transcriptions with written accounts. In a few other cases recordings were not successful for technical reasons and the editor constructed the histories from the questionnaires and interviews. In the text, quotation marks indicate actual spoken words.

A medical career has been described as constantly navigating white water. If that appeals to you, read on...

Further information about the Medical Women's Federation can be obtained from:
The Secretary, Tavistock House North,
Tavistock Square, London WC1H 9HX
Tel/Fax: 020 7387 7765
Email: mwf@btconnect.com . Web page: www.mwfonline.org.uk

ACKNOWLEDGEMENTS

The project was suggested by Dr Mollie McBride, former Honorary Secretary of the Medical Women's Federation.

Financial support was obtained from the Millennium Festival Awards for All programme.

I would like to express my gratitude to all of the following, without whom this book would never have been completed:

> The doctors who so kindly agreed to share their wisdom and experience by taking part in the project, especially Dr Mary Anderson who not only gave her own contribution but also interviewed three other participants for me, and helped with proofreading.
>
> Mr Peter Webster, Head of Personal and Social Health Development at Stockport School, for his encouragement and support in the role of our patron.
>
> Miss Janet Latham, audio-typist, for her expertise and enthusiasm in deciphering the tapes.
>
> My husband Garry for his support and for letting me monopolise the computer.
>
> Our daughters Sophie and Anna who are my inspiration.

Mary Hambleton
September 2001

DR. JOAN WRAY
Pre-NHS General Practitioner

Joan was born on 2nd March 1908 and is our oldest participant. She qualified at the Royal Free in 1932. In her decision to study medicine, like her brother Jack she was strongly influenced by their father, himself a doctor.

She attended St. Paul's Girls' School in London, where the plan to read medicine was considered revolutionary. Music was taught by the composer Gustav Holst, engendering Joan's love of choral singing. Holst's daughter Imogen who was a fellow-pupil became a lifelong friend. Ralph Vaughan Williams also helped teach music in the school.

After qualifying, Joan found hospital appointments without difficulty (but cannot remember where). She married fellow-doctor George in 1936 and they set up in general practice together in Birmingham. She carried this on single-handed when George was abroad in the army during the war with only occasional short periods of leave. This must have been a most difficult time as she had twins in 1941 who both died, one at birth and the other at two weeks. Only eleven months later a son, little George, was born. Employing a nanny, Joan carried on working until the end of the war then, like many other women, gave it up when her husband came back. Another son, John, was born in 1946 and finally a daughter, Mary, in 1948.

It was Mary who revealed that her mother never returned to work after completing her family, explaining why she could say that she did not much notice the advent of the NHS. By then they had moved to Alderley Edge, she must have been wholly taken up with her children at that time and George had begun working in the Prison Service so would be unaffected.

Joan remains reticent about her medical career and has always shown such lively, informed interest in medical matters that one would never suspect she had stopped working before she was forty. She was already seventy when she joined the Medical Women's Federation and merely stated that she had retired.

She nursed George with skill and devotion in his final illness until his death in 1999 and now lives in a residential home. None of her children followed her into medicine but she is delighted that her grandson Jeremy is now a medical student in Nottingham.

DR. SUSANNE LEMPERT-BARBER
Geriatrician

Susi qualified in 1941 at Manchester University; however England was not her native land.

"I come from Holland although I was born in Germany. I spent half my schooling in Holland – finishing at the German School in the Hague which I must say was very nice to start with. It was an international school. The Hague is a place where all the embassies are. And they sent their children to the German School rather than to a Dutch school. But they all left when Hitler came to power. It all changed. I was left, one of the very few Jewish children there. I had a very unpleasant time because the Germans particularly (I don't know about other nations) were more nationalistic outside Germany than they were inside.

"The place was taken over by Nazis. I had two or three very good friends in the class and I stayed in the house of the director who was not a Nazi. When I finished I came to England. I knew I could not study in Germany, and because I had been to a German school I could not study in Holland unless I took their exams. So my father decided I should go to England. In September 1934, I somehow arrived at Reading University, where the term was just about to start. It was very helpful to be there because I could hardly speak English. This was a residential university and you had to speak English all day long.

"It was my own decision to study medicine, but definitely as second choice. My first choice would have been German literature and philosophy, but that was impossible for me to do; so as a second choice I said I wouldn't mind being a doctor. Reading was not a medical school but I could do the pre-medical science subjects there. I took my BSc. Inter exam – botany, zoology, physics and chemistry. My parents encouraged me, and there were some doctors in the family – uncles and so on."

Manchester was not Susi's first choice of medical school.

"It's a long story. In my first year in Reading, my zoology professor had asked me to do some translations from Old Dutch into English. (van Leuwenhoek – you remember). Then he asked me what I was going to do. When I replied I would like to study medicine he said 'Oh, the best medicine is in Edinburgh, and I will speak to my friend the dean of the Faculty there.' So he did and I was offered a place, a year off because I was doing the Inter-Science, and I was working very hard to do the exams because my English was not so good. But in the middle of the exams I get a letter from Edinburgh to say they have so many British people applying to medical school that they can't take me – as an alien. So I was stuck. I wrote to every medical school in the British Isles. The only one to offer me a place was Belfast, but my Father said 'You don't go to Belfast. There is always trouble'. So I stayed in Reading another year. I got in touch through friends of my parents with a lady who worked with the Joint Matriculation Board in Manchester. She told me to apply but that I would have to have Latin. I got on with my studies and also Latin and they accepted me. I had to come to Manchester to take the exam at the College of Preceptors, and they let me off the first MB. I started medical school in October 1936. I stayed at Ashburn Hall which was a huge place. I met several people I'm still friendly with. One of them is Mary Huddert, Mary Wade. She was also doing medicine.

"I must tell you a little bit about the period, because it was 1936-37. Ashburn Hall had several German students there. But they had been sent by the Nazis for propaganda purposes. My friends in Ashburn Hall couldn't understand why I didn't wish to see them. That is just by the way. The senior student there was also a Jewish refugee from Germany – Dr Bergheimer. She had practically finished her studies in Germany, but now had to do it all over again. She eventually became a GP in Middlewich and later in Crewe."

Susi has never wished she had been at a different medical school.

"I was very happy here. I also met my future husband – very quickly – at the fresher's dance. We got married as students. He became a doctor too. (He finally became Assistant Director of clinical pathology at the Manchester Royal Infirmary, and wrote papers on many subjects including haematology). My fiancé was 10 years older than myself, because he had had to support his widowed mother and three other children. He was a scientist, with an MSc in organic chemistry. Now he wanted to start medicine but he could only study medicine part-time; paying his way by working in the lab at the Jewish Hospital. He was a year below me at medical school.

"I'll tell you why we got married so quickly. By now my parents had taken Dutch nationality, but I still had a German passport; and of course I used to visit them quite a lot in the holidays. In 1939, Easter, my father rang up to ask what the political situation was in England, because in Holland they were very scared that the war would start when Mussolini marched into Albania. It was Easter and I was supposed to go over to Holland to my parents. I didn't have a phone but my future husband – to whom I'd got engaged – did have a phone. My father rang him on Good Friday to say he was frightened if I came I wouldn't be allowed back into England. My fiancé told me, 'Your father has just rung up. And he says it's about time you got rid of that German passport', (which of course was nothing like what had been said), 'So I think we'd better get married by special licence.' Which we did, at Bury Register Office. We didn't tell anybody, only two doctor friends of his as witnesses, and we just pretended we were going to the MRI. I was 22."

We might consider that very brave but Susi does not agree.

"No, not at all. But you haven't heard the consequences yet. Next day we went off to Liverpool to get an English passport – instead of the little grey alien's book. So this is 1939 Easter. All went well for a few days and then my mother-in-law – she was very orthodox Jewish – found out about it. And she was absolutely horrified. She threw him out, and me too I suppose. So my father had to come over to help. He was always a very diplomatic person. He explained to her why, and said he would make a proper Jewish wedding any time she liked. It was Passover and it turned out there was an eight week period when you are not allowed to get married. But in the middle of that period there was one day when you are allowed to get married. So we were married on that day. I won't tell you about the wedding. It was very funny but that doesn't matter. So I got married and became British – that's the main thing."

Before long Britain was at war and eventually the Blitz hit Manchester.

"So we carried on with our studies, and when the war started we lived in a flat in Didsbury and even had a refugee girl staying to help us. By chance we were away in the Lake District for a short holiday but came back to the devastation after the bombing. After this Blitz on Manchester our help disappeared She was so terrified she went to live in Buxton. We both moved into Lister House – two little separate rooms. This was the beginning of 1941 – and I worked very hard for my finals. When I qualified I applied to the Infirmary for a house job.

"We were altogether 23 candidates for 22 jobs. We were all paraded round and asked questions. Then 'Daddy' Holmes, (the consultant who had been bombed out and also lived in Lister House at the time), came to me and said, 'You are the only one who has not got a job; you'd better disappear.' I was pretty miserable. But in the middle of dinner I was called to the telephone. A voice said, 'This is Jeffrey Jefferson speaking.' (This was the famous neurosurgeon; he had a funny way of talking, very slow and deliberate.) 'What happened to you?' I said I was the only one without a house job and had been told to go. He said, 'Would you like to work for me?' I said, 'In what capacity?' I thought I was going to wash his boots. Of course I didn't really believe it. I thought it was someone impersonating him. But next morning I went to see him and it was all confirmed. He needed a second houseman. It was a marvellous time and I enjoyed it very much but we worked terribly hard. Sometimes we were six consecutive nights on call. We also never had any meals with anybody else. The Mess at the MRI was still separated. The women were in a little room. There were very few women – perhaps six of us. I remember Olive, who became Olive Nicholson, when she married the surgeon Alan Nicholson. She was a very nice person. Also the women were billeted separately, miles away. I don't remember which part of the hospital but when you were called out at night it took ages to get to the wards.

"After a few months I fell suddenly ill and they put me in a side ward. I was vomiting all the time. People came and examined me. They said, 'It's just D&V', but I kept telling them I didn't have any 'D.' I was saved by another patient coming into this side room. The physician Dr Oliver came to see this patient, but then noticed me and asked me why I was there. He examined me properly and asked could I be pregnant but I said no. He asked for a Gynecology opinion and I had an ovarian cyst removed.

"Then where could I go for convalescence? My husband was still living in just a tiny room in Lister House. 'Daddy' Holmes who was in charge of us said he knew a nice place in the Dales near Bakewell where a retired policeman and his wife had a restaurant and took in people. So he took me there and I had a very pleasant convalescence. Apart from the fact that I got very constipated. You see they kept a turkey. It guarded the outside lavatory and I was too terrified to go.

"Back in Manchester I returned to work with Jefferson, but after a year I got myself a similar job in Sheffield with one of his pupils, the neurosurgeon Mr Harding. He was in charge of the huge head injury centre for servicemen at Fulwood. There was also a surgical ward. I remember a tragic case in the hospital – nothing to do with me. The surgical houseman was supposed to have an appendicectomy. But the general surgeon who operated on him tried to do a very small incision. He did not do his usual routine. He did not look around for the Meckel's diverticulum and missed it. The houseman died. It was before penicillin. He got all the complications – volvulus, gangrene, everything. It was terribly upsetting.

"Most of the young men doctors were by now in the army so we worked terribly hard. Just the consultant and me, living in. I never had a half day. I did everything – house officer cum registrar cum everything.

"I soon realised I was pregnant but kept on working until the end – the ninth month. I went to St Mary's Hospital and saw my friend Kate Liebert who was in charge of me. She examined me and decided it was a breech. She turned it, but when I went back it was again a breech. So they decided I should have an X-ray. At that time St Mary's and MRI had the same X-ray department and I was very well known there because of my many visits as a houseman with encephalograms and ventriculograms and so on. So I saw my own X-ray first. They showed me the films and I realised, before anybody else had seen it, that it was anencephalic. It is a very strange thing, and that's why I mention it. You recognise it and yet you don't take it in. Everyone was very upset. I was induced but the baby didn't live.

"After that I must have gone back to work for Jefferson, mainly outpatients but also assisting at operations. The next year we had our first daughter. My husband was still doing his house jobs at the time, but he was about to join the Airforce and went to India. So I was left living with the baby in an upstairs flat.

"My husband had only just arrived in India, (I had had a letter from him), when I received a telegram from the Air Ministry to say that they regret to inform me that my husband is dangerously ill and they will let me know when they know more. Well, I don't think they ever did tell me he was out of danger! I was terribly worried. What happened was that he had both amoebic and bacillary dysentery at the same time. He diagnosed himself because nobody else could. He was supposed to set up a pathology lab in the place, but illness had overtaken him. When his high fever had come down he was able to do his own lab tests.

"When he felt better they sent him into the mountains and he had a wonderful time. He took some superb photographs of it all – he was a very keen photographer. When he finally came home he was still being treated by the RAF over here. I stayed working for Jefferson. In 1947 we had our second daughter.

"Has coping with home and children been difficult to fit in with work? I must say that I worked all my life until 65, mostly part-time once we had the children. You can't do everything. We had a mother's help and a charwoman. I did not take much time off after giving birth. My children sometimes said things – about how lovely it was at a friend's house with a mother always at home and doing the baking."

Susi's career path had many twists and turns.

"I was still with Jefferson but about the fifth wheel on the ladder. I didn't want to work all the time, so I tried some general practice locums, but then decided 'No. I'll do my DPH' (Diploma of Public Health). This was a very interesting period because they had just appointed a Professor of Social and Preventive Medicine. He was running the course, and it was completely new. We learnt amazing subjects; Social Anthropology, Genetics, Bacteriology of course, Sociology, Social Administration. All sorts of things. It was a marvellous course. If someone had come to us and said 'You have to learn Chinese' we would have thought, 'Yes, that belongs in Social and Preventive Medicine too.' The professor, Fraser Brockington, was and is a most interesting person, but always away and writing books. He is still alive, and still writes to me at Christmas. He attracted the most interesting people, the foremost people in their fields, as lecturers. It was the time when a lot of doctors were leaving South Africa. The department was almost taken over by South Africans.

"Afterwards I did a locum in public health – in Hyde, I remember. (I don't remember Dr Shipman – I suppose he wasn't there yet). It was in public health that I saw the other side of neurosurgery – remaining disabilities and how to deal with them in the community. I was asked to do a survey of old people in Stockport. This came under our Department of Social and Preventive Medicine. I was very interested in that. I looked only at the over-eighties – the questions about their social status, what they did and so on. I had to give them a report. I was invited to the Town Hall – it was all very festive. And later on I wrote a book about it: 'The Social Needs of the Over Eighties.'

"But in the middle of all this, after I had finished the practical work, my husband died – on the golf course of all places. I just didn't want to be bothered with all those ciphers and figures and so on. Later I wrote it all up and there were some papers published, but for now I wanted to be back in medicine; proper medicine. But I finished the book, which I wrote with Professor Brockington. Of course he had to be in on it. Which was all very nice because I had suggested that there should be Geriatric Units. There were very few Geriatric Units in those days, but by the time I came to be employed as a geriatrician there was a unit in Stockport, and they asked me to be their first registrar. In the meantime of course I was trying to get the Membership.

"Now we come to the last period of my medical career. I became a geriatrician. I worked first at Stockport. Then the geriatrician from Withington came to ask me to come to Withington. They were about to appoint a professor of geriatrics. So I went to Withington and when the professor was appointed I also got a sort of assistant lectureship. I was more interested in research. So I later on did a big research programme together with the Geriatric Unit in London – Professor Exton-Smith was his name. It was a two-town survey of fractured femurs. I looked at all the fractured femurs from the orthopaedic departments of Withington, the MRI and Wythenshawe. And the London people doing theirs. We wrote several papers, and I also wrote up the Stockport survey – and got married to my second husband.

"In the last few years of my working life I took on the day hospital in Stockport. You can do such a lot with a day hospital. The patients don't have to get lost on a ward. You can treat them very well. You can do almost everything in a day hospital for old people.

"I don't remember healthcare before the NHS …yes I do. I remember we were all very pro-NHS when it was coming in. But now we have seen it gradually decline. Even when I was still working it deteriorated terribly."

Susi remembers using M&B (a sulphonamide) when she was doing neurosurgery but penicillin was not introduced until she was in public health.

"Our daughter fell ill when she was five, with otitis media. The paediatrician sent her to a female ENT specialist who admitted her to Pendlebury Hospital for a myringotomy. (In those days children in hospital, and their parents, had a very raw deal. I wrote about it afterwards.) It would not heal. My husband suggested he could get some penicillin for her, but the consultant said it would cover up or conceal any complications. We didn't dare argue. Our child was very unhappy. Visiting was only once a week and when we came to see her she cried and cried and wouldn't settle. In the end they reluctantly said you'd better come every day. The wards were very long and she was right at the other end. There was an antediluvian trolley coming down the ward, creaking, never oiled, slowly coming nearer – like a horror film. She was terrified. I was sent out while two people held her down and poked in her ear. It was like torture. After that I said I would like to take her home. So we did. Our own GP got us some penicillin powder which we put in, and it all cleared up. But my poor daughter was maimed for life – not physically. She became very quiet, and so on. For the DPH you had to write a dissertation, so I wrote mine on children in hospital. I did research for it at Booth Hall. Later it all changed. You remember someone wrote a book, and there was the film of what happens to children. But that was our experience of children in hospital."

Susi would not, with hindsight, have changed the timing of her family. "…because my husband was older than me. He was well into his thirties, and then he died in his early fifties."

Career decisions were made as she went along.

"Well, there are deciding moments. There is a word for this in German – 'Star times'. One such moment was when I was offered the post of Chief Assistant in Neurosurgery. I turned it down. You are not there on your own. Another moment was with my second husband. I was in the middle of taking Membership. He didn't stop me, in fact he was very encouraging, but I decided not. You can only go so far and then you have to consider other people. You may always be sorry in some way, but you have to make sacrifices particularly as a woman. There are always family problems in any job."

Both daughters have gone into professions allied to medicine.

"One is a speech therapist and one a social worker. That one developed Temporal Lobe Epilepsy – after she was married. It has prevented her from getting jobs – even though she only gets a few little absences and occasional episodes of slight automatism. So you see Social Services do not practise what they preach.

"How do I rate the contribution of women doctors? No different from men, though they have to balance many more things."

Susi was an active member of MWF for many years.

"Oh, I did quite a bit. I was on the Council, and then Local President when the AGM was held here in Manchester… like you have just done this year. Great fun and very necessary, then – and probably still is.

"I retired in 1980 at the age of 65 having always worked until then. That felt very nice. We started a completely different life. At first I tried a course in Archaeology, but the physical work of digging in Wales in the rain was too much for me. Then we started English literature from the beginning, at the extramural department. Beowulf onwards. You know as doctors we don't read much, do we? Sadly my husband died in April 2000. They looked after him – us – very well. In the autumn I will get a Hallé season ticket, but I do not like to go alone. My daughters come up. We go shopping and have been to the theatre.

"What advice would I offer to young people contemplating medicine as a career? I am not sure – I have been out of it for too long. Everyone seems fed up with it, not enough beds, not enough staff. I know medicine had to change from being too jolly and paternalistic, but what has replaced it? Too many managers. I know a number of colleagues have advised their children NOT to do medicine. I think that is sad."

DR. MARGARET JESSUP
General Practitioner

Dr Jessup died on 6th December 2000, aged 75. A member of MWF for 33 years and Past President of Manchester Association, she made this contribution for our Millennium Project on 25th May 2000. The passages in quotes are her own words recorded on tape. Her enthusiasm and humour shine through even though she was already on chemotherapy at that time. We offer deepest sympathy to her husband Geoffrey and the children, Christine, Susan, Anne, John and Peter.

Margaret qualified at Manchester University in 1949. There were no other doctors in her family. It was her own decision to study medicine and she experienced some discouragement about this at school.

"I remember my Headmistress saying, 'Oh, it's not a job for a woman. You could be a hospital almoner because you could put the instruments out for the surgeon.' That just shows how little they knew about things in those days. I had a German teacher who was a German refugee in this country, of course this was in 1942, and she said, 'Oh Margaret, I don't think you should do medicine because you know there are times in the month when a woman isn't at her best.' Then of course the main difficulty I had was that I liked biology very much and I had a wonderful teacher who lent me a great tome on bacteriology and I was fascinated by it. She was lovely, she was great, but I decided that the only way to become a bacteriologist would be to do a degree in science and get a 1st Class and then be able to do research, and I thought I wasn't 1st class honours material so I abandoned that and then to my horror when I did apply for medicine at University, I found that I needed physics and chemistry and I had not done physics and chemistry, maybe I'd done a bit of chemistry but certainly no physics at school certificate which I took in 1940. I changed school because of the war; I went back to North Wales where it was considered safe. In order to do physics and chemistry I did school certificate physics and chemistry in one year, we did what were called supplementary subjects and then I attempted to do higher school certificate physics and chemistry which I hadn't got any grounding in and never understood. The worst exam I've ever taken was my practical physics. I had to go down to Barmouth Grammar School from Dolgellau to take it and I was presented with this Wheatstone bridge and I didn't know what it was for or which end was which, it was terrible.

"I had applied for Manchester and Leeds because university entrance was zoned in those war years; because my home was in Blackburn, I could only apply for Manchester, Leeds, Liverpool, Sheffield or Birmingham, which were the five northern universities, and I went for an interview to Leeds. Both Leeds and Manchester were very keen on medical students having an arts subject as well as science and Leeds gave me a provisional acceptance as long as I got physics and chemistry at Higher School Certificate with my English literature. Manchester accepted me unconditionally. I got into Manchester on a load of these supplementary subjects. All my usual matric. subjects plus physics and chemistry and I'd done German because I thought it might be useful for bacteriology or science or something, all at what would be called O-level now and I got in on subsidiary Higher School Certificate in English literature. The other reason that I got in was that from my school, Dr Williams School, Dolgellau, I was the fourth girl in succession to go to Manchester Medical School. They obviously liked our school and they took girls from Dr Williams School. So I had problems with 1st MB with my physics, chemistry was all right, and after a cramming course took 1st MB again and passed.

"So I then set off on my anatomy and everything else and never looked back. I chose medicine because I liked people and as I got on with it I thought I would like to be a medical missionary because the church I belonged to, which was then the Congregational Church, ran the London Missionary Society that had sent out David Livingstone many years ago. Howard Somervell, who went up Everest in the 1924 expedition with Mallory and Irving, visited Manchester and explained the need for medical services in South India, where he founded a hospital and training college still in existence today. In those days there was a very strong missionary influence on young people my age."

Margaret's eventual career was the result of seizing opportunity.

"I still had this idea of being a medical missionary, of course in those days you got your house jobs to get the experience because you learnt a lot from them. I did a student locum on M3 at MRI and Dr William Brockbank who was the consultant in charge (he died some years ago) said to me one day, 'When you qualify which job would you like?' Well, I'd have been a fool, wouldn't I, not to say, 'This one.' He said okay and the way we got jobs then was we all piled into the boardroom at the MRI and they read out the list of consultants and they read the name of the person who was going to work with them, you see, so I set off on that. My senior registrar when I was at MRI was Richard Stone who was very young when he got his job as a consultant at the Northern Hospital, he was 32. Perhaps they get them now, but that was the minimum age for a consultant in those days. He was a general physician and he rang up and said, 'Get your hat on and get up here for the interviews.' Again it's a useful reflection that you were supposed to, you know, you wore a suitable suit and you put your hat on and I went up for the interview, and of course I got the job which was a bit hard on the other girl at the time because she'd done a locum there, but anyway Richard must have thought I was worth having. Then after that I got a surgical job at the Northern Hospital. That was a very useful job, because with only five residents there was opportunity for wide experience in general surgery, ENT, gynaecology, general medicine and paediatrics.

"Meanwhile Geoff was working at Withington and at Ancoats; he was RCO at Ancoats for a bit and clinical pathologist at Withington and we got married about 18 months after qualifying, when we'd got any money to get married on, and I went to do a midwifery job at Crumpsall, again to get midwifery experience, then I found I was pregnant which was a big surprise to me. As regards planning your family, there was very little planning in those days, mostly caps, you know, it wasn't very much. I never thought I'd get pregnant so soon because I'd always had frequent amenorrhoea, I had three months of amenorrhoea just for doing finals so I was very surprised, I was very overjoyed and she's 48 this year. So anyway I stopped work when I had Christine and there was never any question of having any money to pay for au pairs, no child help at all so I only did locums more to help to pay the mortgage than anything. I learned quite a bit of general practice that way, which was a bit hard on the patients probably, but I worked as a locum for very good, kind GPs, one was Muriel Edwards and also Winifred Hall. Both have died now, they were in Northenden. They were very kind to me and taught me a lot. I did that until the youngest of our five children started school in 1966 when the new Group Practice Allowance was introduced to encourage GPs to work in groups of three or more. This was the government policy – they didn't like single-handed practitioners and they said that if you had three partners, you got a financial incentive.

"I was in practice for 20 years, I was 40 when I went back to work because my husband's senior partner retired. He was only 46 but he hated the health service, in fact he didn't like medicine at all, so when he had been in the health service for 10 years he was able to retire. My husband and his remaining partner decided to take their wives in and they thought we'd be okay for locums or something like that and they weren't very helpful. I remember the other man saying once to his wife when she and I were talking, "Come on girls, stop chatting, get on with the work," and what we were discussing was the patients we'd seen in surgery and the patients we were going to go out and see and looking at the records, looking things up. Jean did school clinics, and she'd also done occasional surgeries with children and in the practice and then she had two children. Anyway we got our foot well and truly in, and of course like all partners in practice we thought we did more work than they did. I attended a lot of postgraduate revision courses at weekends and lunchtimes and successfully took the examinations for MRCGP (Member of the Royal College of General Practitioners).

"My husband was a Course Organiser, he started the first Vocational Training Course in General Practice in South Manchester, in Wythenshawe, when these Vocational Training Courses were coming in, so he was out and about on Wednesday for day release and the other male partner went to play golf, so Jean and I ran the practice that day. I loved working in Wythenshawe. So I started when I was 40 and I resigned at 60, and I did family planning at the same time and did my family planning certificate, of course, when I was in practice because Jean and I did most of that. Geoff used to do cytology, (smears), and he did a lot of ante-natals too. Some people, even when I was there, would prefer to go to him. There are some patients who think a man is a proper doctor. Of course he was very gentle, very nice.

"When I was 60 I left General Practice because it was full time, I mean we did weekends and nights. Although there were four of us we were two couples, so obviously when Geoff was on I answered the phone as well, you know, all the calls came through to us, so we did alternate weekends and when the other two went on holiday we doubled up, we had six weeks holiday a year and the six weeks were split into two lots of three, whenever we had our summer holiday with our children our partners did all the work, we never had locums, we just doubled up and we could manage. So then I went on… well, I didn't plan to do full time family planning, but I did because people knew me and I was known at Palatine Road FP Centre. So I worked for North, Central and South Manchester and also got onto Trafford because I'd moved here (to Bowdon) so was in Trafford. I did a lot of family planning everywhere until I was 65 and I thought they'd throw me out then, so I finished."

Margaret counted qualifying as a doctor and obtaining a GP partnership as the professional achievements which pleased her most. The greatest challenge was balancing loyalties to practice and family. In her time she was active on medical committees such as the LMC, FPC and service committees. Her many other interests included religion, music and the arts. After retiring she obtained an Open University BA degree in Arts Subjects. Margaret rated the NHS as excellent from her own experience, though aware that not everyone would agree. She considered the greatest challenge in the future will be to maintain good doctor-patient relationships in spite of bureaucracy. Although none of her children have gone into medicine Margaret would encourage young people to "Go for it!" – but to aim always for high standards and job satisfaction regardless of financial benefits.

DR. KATIE WHALE
Microbiologist

Katie qualified in 1955 at Manchester Medical School, which was her first choice and one which she has never regretted. Her school, in the state system, was not encouraging about her ambition to study medicine but her parents were on her side, even though there were no other doctors in the family.

After qualifying she did not experience any difficulty in obtaining posts but her career path was influenced by her domestic situation. She got married two years before finals and bore her only child two years after qualifying, returning to work within a month. Baby Zoë was cared for by a childminder for her first five months and subsequently went to a council day-nursery. When Katie's husband was away on business and she was on call, she would have the baby with her in the hospital overnight, relying on staff to help out, then would rush off with the pram to the nursery a mile away, returning in time for the 8.30 theatre list.

"On the question of career paths, I quite by accident got into respiratory medicine. The plot was initially to do pathology, and I had actually applied for a post with the Public Health Laboratory in 1958 just after the birth of my daughter who was born in August 1957. But it quickly became apparent, the Public Health Laboratory being based in Monsall at the time, that I would have a hell of a job getting from South Manchester over to North Manchester with a small baby. It so happened that I had been SHO in pathology at Wythenshawe Hospital and had had my baby given a BCG vaccination in preparation for my supposed post with the Public Health Laboratory and of course she developed a BCG abscess. So I went off to the Baguley Chest Clinic and was seen by the consultant physician there, Tom Wilson, who said, 'We will treat that with isoniazid and would you like a job?' so I said, 'OK.' And that was really how I entered chest medicine, quite by chance.

"After 15 years I had become increasingly interested in opportunist pulmonary infections, particularly fungal infections, and as there was nobody at that time in the North West doing any mycology of pulmonary infections at all, I decided I would go and do that, but it meant retraining in microbiology. So I switched over to microbiology in 1973 and of course had to retrain completely and eventually gained my MRCPath in 1977. I was appointed as Consultant Medical Microbiologist in North Manchester in 1980. At that time I had already established a small working laboratory for the diagnosis of fungal infection – systemic, pulmonary fungal infection – and I continued that work in North Manchester. So essentially I became the mycology guru for the Northwest and I continued that work until I retired in 1990.

"The question of coping with home and children and this difficulty of fitting in work, it's a difficult one to answer. I wouldn't say it's been difficult, just not easy at times, the question is juggling all one's responsibilities to husband, to child, to home, to job, to oneself, particularly I guess to oneself. I think it's probably the one aspect of my daughter's work [nursing] that I've been keen to emphasise for her that whatever she does she must make time for herself, for her own mental well-being and, as a knock-on-effect, that of her children and her partner. Also I think it's very important to keep up outside interests, we've all seen colleagues who seem to be totally engrossed in their work, who seem to be really less satisfactory characters as a result of that. Not having any outside interests seems to me to have a very bad effect on the human being and in particular with their relationship to society as a whole."

Katie says the professional achievement which pleased her most was getting her MRCPath. She does not recall any major disappointments. The greatest challenge she had to meet was dealing with infectious diseases physicians.

"I made the comment about greatest professional challenge, about the infectious diseases physicians; it's not entirely tongue in cheek actually. I had a great deal of difficulty when I was appointed consultant in North Manchester, not from any of the other clinicians, but specifically from infectious diseases physicians and this was really because they viewed themselves as their own microbiologists and felt that they were the ones who would decide how the laboratory would be used. Unfortunately they met with me, who had very firm ideas about running a laboratory because of my excellent training both in Public Health and at Withington Microbiology Department, so there was not just clash of personalities but a clash of ethos and I was determined to win.

"How do I rate the NHS? Well that's very hard to say. I'm fortunate in that by and large I've really not had to use its services. It seems to me however, sadly, that for whatever reason, and you can postulate quite a few, there are now so many delays in providing a service that in fact it would appear that most services now can only be described as second rate, if not third rate. The problem is that it's not just a medical problem, though. There's the problem of other kinds of care as well, particularly nursing care and I think it's those aspects that particularly worry me when seeing friends and relatives in hospital, for there almost seems to be a culture of neglect which I find absolutely appalling. And it's not because the nurses are less intelligent nor do I think it's necessarily that they've got more form filling or bureaucracy to contend with. Whether or not it's a question of demoralisation I just don't know, but these girls come into nursing with a vocation and yet it seems that in a very short time they just become non-thinking, non-interested people who really don't give any quality of service at all, that's not to say they all do, obviously, but this is an overall appearance it seems to me.

"My advice to any young person contemplating a career in medicine would be 'Go for it!'"

And there is life after medicine: since retirement Katie has taken a first-class BA degree and BPhil. in the History of Art and has been commissioned to make a catalogue of the mediaeval stained glass (up to 1550) of Cheshire, Greater Manchester and Merseyside. She continues her active interest in the theatre and music including an annual visit to the Aldeburgh Festival.

DR. RAINE ROBERTS
General Practitioner and Clinical Forensic Specialist

"I qualified at Manchester University in 1955. This medical school was my first choice though when I was a child, I had thoughts that I might go to Edinburgh or Aberdeen but I didn't even apply there. I haven't wished that I'd been at a different university. I do think Manchester University in the 1950's was one of the best in Europe.

"I was firmly of the opinion for a very long time that it was my own decision to study medicine but when I was little I wanted to be a teacher and it was my mother who put the idea into my head that I ought to be a doctor. She was a very intelligent woman who went to school from the age of nine until the age of thirteen, two of those years were spent teaching the younger children, and she never had the opportunity to benefit from higher education. My parents were farmers and it was my mother who was very ambitious and wanted me not to have all the hassle of getting up to milk the cows and working seven days a week, and for goodness sake I'm nearly seventy and I'm still getting up and working seven days a week! There were no other doctors in our family, I was the first and the only member of my family to go to university and was something of a phenomenon in the family because I used to be able to pass exams. I was very greatly encouraged by my mother who was the ambitious one and my father fully supported his bright little daughter doing well at the high school. The school was very supportive and it was a single-sex school that encouraged the girls to do what they could. The only discouragement I ever got, which was amusing really, was a man in the village where our farm was said to my father when I was about sixteen, 'Fancy keeping that lass at school when she could be at t'mill earning £6 a week.' The mill is no longer there and the mill workers aren't earning anything so here we are. That was other peoples' attitudes, not my family's. My school was the local high school; I passed the exam to get in there – Burnley High School.

"After qualifying, I didn't have any difficulty in obtaining posts. I had house jobs at Manchester Royal Infirmary. I worked for Professor later Lord Platt, President of the Royal College of Physicians, and in the neurosurgical department and then in paediatrics. I worked mainly in general practice for about thirty years and latterly in clinical forensic medicine, particularly in the fields of sexual assault and child abuse. I think my eventual career path was a matter of making a decision. I met a tall, dark and handsome medical student on the first day I came to Manchester University and I think in those days if I'd have wanted to be a consultant physician I felt I would have to have been single-mindedly pursuing that line, and might see myself in an elegant flat at the age of fifty on my own, or I could marry this very dishy chap that I fancied and bring up a family and go into general practice with him. Our idea was that we would go into a little country practice, a little country town. We ended up staying in Manchester for the next thirty years. Really because the practice came along which was ideally suited to us in that a single-handed practitioner was going to retire and leave the north of England, so my husband would be his own boss at the age of about thirty and that suited him very well. So we worked together in those days, he ran the practice, and I did some work and brought up the children. I never changed my mind about what I wanted to do, that was it, I made a decision – was I going to go into hospital medicine and work really hard and single-mindedly at that, or do what I did.

"We got married as students when both of us had passed second MB, it took my husband longer than me because he'd done Arts at school and had been in the army as an Army officer and had to learn Science really from square one, so that it took him a bit longer, but when we both got second MB we got married and we have been in practice for the whole of our professional lives.

"I have two children, my daughter was born in 1960 and my son in 1962 and yes, they were planned and I think it worked out very well. My husband had gone into the practice and I was working as a registrar in Blackburn. The first pregnancy came at the end of my registrar job and I sat there whilst Jim was doing the practice and then went into the practice after the first child was born, so that seemed to work out very well. The time I took off after giving birth, as I say I'd left my registrar job and I wasn't then a partner in the practice, I used to do odd bits of surgeries for other doctors a few weeks after having the children, and then when the second one was born I was a partner, and I just had a very short time off and started doing a few surgeries again.

"Coping with home and children has worked very well because we've lived in a house which is next door to where the practice was running, and I've always had very good home help support and, most importantly, the full support of my husband. It was nice that we had our surgery in the house next door because we could have a coffee with the children and my daughter, particularly, would like to come and do the follow-up visits to the old ladies and they would like to see the doctor's little girl. The childcare, I've had good childcare. I had a Princess Christian trained nanny who used to come in part-time and I'd come out of the surgery, she would be under the dining table with sheets and curtains in this den with my children, and that was really good. Both my children are now doctors, my daughter was a GP partner in Windsor but she is now married to an American surgeon, lives in the mid-west of America and does now practice in Family Medicine, having had to convince the Americans that she was a doctor in spite of having her MRCGP and everything that you could require to be a good GP. My son, the younger one, is a consultant orthopaedic surgeon at the Robert Jones and Agnes Hunt Hospital at Oswestry and at Wrexham.

"My principal outside interests are gardening, admiring the three grandchildren and water-skiing at Sale Water Park, which I still do, perhaps foolishly, but it does blow the cobwebs away.

"What's the greatest professional challenge I've had to meet? I think this was the Cleveland matter, it was a really enormous event both nationally and for the medical profession which didn't exactly cover itself with glory. The Butler-Sloss Inquiry criticised everybody in sight including me which I thought very unfair and there are many inaccuracies in it, but you have to struggle on. It was certainly an illuminating and learning experience and I honestly did my best to assist the courts, to assist the families and children that I came across, but it wasn't always received with enthusiasm, but there we are.

"I was accused in the Cleveland Inquiry Report of having been biased in favour of the parents and not being objective, and I thought that was grossly unfair because I did in fact put information before the courts and the inquiry that didn't necessarily support the people who'd instructed me. I would go and see children or give reports into court and if I didn't find that I could support what parents were saying then that was clearly said, but it certainly didn't come out in the inquiry and I didn't know I was on trial, but it was certainly an enormous trauma. I don't think anybody who hasn't been through it would realise how traumatic it was.

"What happened was that there was the article in the Lancet about the buggery that came from Leeds, and I wrote a letter to the Lancet saying it didn't accord with my own experience with a large number of children in Manchester over time, and that was that. That was in the November of 1986 and then the Cleveland thing really started hitting the newspapers. My stance was that I've seen a lot of children, I don't see buggery being as common as they say and I don't see this anal sign being terribly reliable. I can't remember what the actual letter said, but because of that, some solicitors in Cleveland asked me to go and do some examinations, which I did and then gave evidence in court where I was actually praised by the judge as being the model of an expert witness, but not by the inquiry. I didn't know what the agenda of the inquiry was but I was very naïve in those days.

"I think the way I got involved in it in the first place was being asked to go and give an expert opinion. I was a GP in Manchester, I did examinations and being asked to go to the Inquiry and all that stuff, you know, I was flattered by that and I didn't realise just how difficult it was. I am more streetwise now of course in this sort of area but you can see how that would happen. I'd written this letter to Lancet and the next thing was, 'Dr Roberts, come up to Middlesborough to do these examinations.' My honest belief about many of the children I examined, and that was only a proportion of them, was that they had not been abused. There was no evidence that they had and that was really quite difficult to cope with and was certainly the biggest professional challenge I've had to meet. Then to have to live afterwards with the fact that I had been criticised in a public document and that if I went into court, for instance, that might well be raised and I would have to deal with it. Interestingly in 1991 I spoke at a symposium at the Royal College of Physicians on the same platform as Lady Butler-Sloss, and in the meantime both of us I think had learnt quite a lot.

"I think my best professional achievement was being involved in setting up the St. Mary's Centre, which does provide a good service to the people of Manchester who have the misfortune to suffer sexual assault."

Many MWF members remember the Manchester AGM in the early 1980's when Doctor Roberts launched the idea of a Sexual Assault Referral Centre in response to concerns about lack of facilities in those days and the way women were treated. A Working Group was set up as a direct result of that lecture with Police, Doctors and Hospital Managers working together to set up the St. Mary's Centre, which opened in 1986. It is a collaborative venture between Greater Manchester Police and the Central Manchester Healthcare NHS Trust. It offers a comprehensive and coordinated forensic examination, counselling and medical aftercare service to adults who have been raped or sexually assaulted. It serves a population of two and a half million and sees about six hundred clients per year, four percent of whom are male. Police referrals make up about two thirds, the other one third are self-referrals. There are separate arrangements for children. In recognition of this work Dr Roberts was awarded the MBE.

"What advice would I offer to young people contemplating medicine as a career? Well, if you must be a doctor just go for it. How do I rate the contribution women doctors can make? What has that got to do with it; if you are a doctor, you are a doctor.

"My greatest disappointment in my career, I think, is the Cleveland thing and being publicly criticised was a terrible disappointment. I felt it was wrong, I felt it was unjust, I still do, but you have to live with it.

"How do I rate the NHS? I used to think it was wonderful and when I was a young doctor I did whatever I thought was right for my patients without thought of the cost, referred wherever I might get the best advice, but you can't always do that now. I had a patient who wanted to be a ballerina, I could send her to the best person, who knew the most about this, at Charing Cross, who looked after the Royal Ballet School. You couldn't do this now without a lot of paperwork and bureaucracy and contracts, etc. The only thing I remember about healthcare before the NHS was having diphtheria at the age of five. I was tied down so that I didn't move or jump about, in case I died of heart failure (that probably scarred me for life). That was quite an experience. Nobody thought of saying anything to the child about why she needed to lie flat.

"What do I regard as the greatest challenge to medicine in the future? Being able to afford everything that can be done, for example I remember a conversation with my son, when he was a medical student, towering over me in the kitchen. We were talking about working all hours in the 50's and he said, 'You may have worked all those hours for your patients but you couldn't actually do anything.' He's wiser now! – of course that's not true, there was a lot we could do and did, we worked very hard and we looked after our patients, but I do remember when working for Lord Platt, a young woman on the ward screaming over and over again, 'I don't want to die, I don't want to die.' She was 21 – a year or two younger than me. These days she would have had a kidney transplant."

MISS CARYS BANNISTER
Neurosurgeon

Carys qualified in 1958 at Charing Cross Hospital Medical School, University of London. Until the age of fifteen she was living in Brazil where her father was working as a railway engineer. She came back to England to finish her education, initially at a private girls' school near Guildford and then at a state technical college. It was her own idea to study medicine. There were no doctors in previous generations in her family but a cousin 3-4 years older than herself was already at medical school in London.

"In answer to the question was my medical school my first choice? No, but in fact I had only just come over from Brazil two years previously and I really didn't know anything about medical schools at all. I was in school in Surrey and in fact the school I was at couldn't do A-levels in all science subjects, so I'd left and gone to the Guildford County Technical College and when I went up to various interviews, my parents had gone back to Brazil and my sister and I couldn't find the medical schools and I went along, I had long hair and socks and honestly I can't blame any medical schools for turning me down and it's all very despairing really. My mum was against medicine, she said it was unladylike, and never did she say a truer word but still... and then she went back to Brazil but she'd persuaded me not to do the right A-levels so I was actually doing pure and applied maths, physics and chemistry. I went to the Head of the Department and said I wanted to do medicine and he said, 'Well, you're doing the wrong A-levels.' They did A-levels in one year at that place so he said to me, 'Oh, it's too late now, you're halfway through the first term, you've only got another two and half terms, you can't possibly change at this stage, so do what you're doing and next year you can do botany and zoology.' So it seemed quite reasonable and as it turned out he advised me well because all these medical schools uniformly had said 'No,' which was no great surprise but the second year he said to me, 'Oh, botany and zoology, you can't do that, it's not enough, you'd better do a State Scholarship,' and I was still absolutely terribly naïve, I didn't know what he was talking about. So I did chemistry at Scholarship level and zoology at Scholarship level and I actually got a State Scholarship, but having applied to all the medical schools again they still all turned me down and so he came round, I always remember, he came round to the house where my sister and I were staying with a housekeeper and he said to me, 'Take this bit of paper and go back to those medical schools again,' and Charing Cross was the one that offered me a place to start in three weeks so I don't know whether that was a choice. I had a cousin who did medicine and he was at the London so I think if I'd have had a free choice in those days, I would probably have chosen the London Hospital. I never thought of going anywhere further because it was such a jolt coming from Brazil and the thought of actually leaving the house where my sister was was too much really, to think of going anywhere else anyway. Nobody ever discussed anywhere else so that's the long answer saying no, but I was very happy there."

Carys made an early decision to go into neurosurgery though this was not an easy path to take. Concerning the question of gender discrimination:

"After qualifying there were no problems during house jobs, but when I applied for an SHO post in Surgery, I applied for a lot of them and in fact the post I was eventually given was on the refusal of somebody else, you know, I was second choice. But I have to say, before that I had gone to the Accident Hospital in Birmingham because at that time you had to do A&E for the Fellowship, you had to have done Casualty and I must admit that at the Accident hospital in Birmingham, although I was the only woman there they were very supportive and I can't say that there were any problems then. The problems came really when I applied for jobs that were above the House Officer level, but in fact after I'd done that SHO post I did the Fellowship and then I went to Oxford and took two and a half years out because I did a BSc. I did a research project in the Department of Physiology and wrote a thesis.

"Up until going to Oxford learning had been cramming, but it was peculiar to my circumstances. I mean I'd come over from Brazil, from an American Graded School. There isn't a great meeting of the ways in American education and British education and when I came I was just fifteen and it was just at the time, it didn't last long actually, when you had to be sixteen to do O-levels, you couldn't do them earlier. It was also a time when you couldn't be graded, you either had to pass or fail. It was one of those passing fancies of the Ministry of Education I suppose, but anyway I had to be crammed because they'd already started all their courses by the time I got into school, so I just had all these tutors and extra lessons and goodness knows what to do these O-levels and I've still no idea what they were about, really. Then I went to the Technical College and, as I say, you did the A-level course in one year. You can imagine how cramming that was, and then you went to medical school and in London you did second

MB in 18 months and then the rest of medicine was crammed into the next three years. There had never been any time to do anything in depth and then going to Oxford suddenly I knew the difference, when I got there, between being taught and educated. It was a complete reopening of my eyes, but it was peculiar to my circumstances and I knew it really when I talked to other people, you know, they were very eloquent in telling me the difference. I mean it was only in Oxford I'd ever heard anyone read poetry, it's amazing, it's very sad really, but there you are, we survived I guess.

"It was very interesting when I think about it, I was so fortunate to be there, but so ignorant, the first three terms I did the ordinary lectures and wrote essays and read them to Jean Bannister and people like Hilary Brown. Because I went with the idea I was determined to do research Jean said to me, 'Oh you should do it with…' I've forgotten the man's name, but he did a lot of transport mechanisms across cell membranes and I said, 'Oh no, I'm not going to do that.' She actually got me to go and see him and I was absolutely determined I wasn't going to do it after seeing him. He was a super man and he was highly intelligent, but it wasn't what I wanted, I wanted to do some physiological experiments that involved animal research. It sounds ironic really because of the way I think of animals, but in fact what I did was intracellular recordings from motor neurones in the spinal cord and looked at the input from stimulation of the pyramidal tract, comparing the input between the upper limb and lower limb motor neurone groups, and it was fiendishly difficult, with a tutor who was an Australian chap called Bob Porter. He was a Rhodes Scholar from Melbourne, and my goodness, he certainly taught me research methods. He was so precise, so harsh, he expected results every week and of course most of the cells went off like whizz-bang rockets and the minute you prodded them they objected, so if you got a cell that was recording you would stay there all night with it, but I was never so pleased as when he said to me, 'I could do the whole of this project in one week.' So I said to him, 'Well, just do one animal,' and he couldn't get a cell! It was so good. I thought, 'This project will work,' and in the end it did after a fashion, but most important it taught me research methods.

"When I came out from Oxford and went to try and find a post in neurosurgery I found some difficulty, in fact I'd done a previous SHO post in Edinburgh and I thought it might be nice to go back and do a registrar post there but they wouldn't have me, but I went to Leeds. The real difficulty came in getting appointed as a consultant, I think compared to men I was delayed, but again I came here to Manchester to do a locum and they virtually created a post for me at North Manchester and Booth Hall Children's Hospital, so in the end I made it, but it was difficult. I went to an awful lot of interviews, in fact so many interviews I lost count and there was a very talented Indian chap, we used to say we were window-dressing, we used to go and have a cup of tea and a sticky bun afterwards, but he was appointed in Newcastle eventually and I was appointed here, so both of us weren't as easy to displace I think as people thought we might be."

Carys still feels it was a disappointment in her career failing to obtain a consultant post in Leeds, where she had worked as a registrar and had already begun work she wished to continue. However she was extremely successful in Manchester. The professional achievement which has pleased her most was obtaining an OBE for her services to neurosurgery in Manchester.

She believes the greatest challenge for medicine in the future will be to get rid of surgery, which is a crude and imprecise method of treatment. She considers that women doctors can make just the same contribution as men, no better and no worse.

Her career has been the most important thing in her life and she has never married, however she is involved with her sister and family. She lives in a charming converted farmhouse above Rawtenstall and looks after a large collection of animals, which are her principal outside interest.

She is not happy about recent developments in the NHS. "I say about the Health Service, 'It's gone to the dogs.' I think the awful thing about the Health Service is that many of the reforms on paper sound absolutely right, don't they? It's so difficult to pick out any particular thing, but take regulation of clinical outcome, it sounds such a good thing, let's improve the standards. How do you improve standards because there isn't, if you look in neurosurgery, there is not a standard way of doing any procedure, it's got to be tailormade to the individual patient. The individual patient has got so many variations and biological differences, I really don't know how you sit down and work out outcome and some of the outcomes are unrealistic. To look at, say, survival at one month, it means nothing. I mean you could make the survival at one month for tumours a lot better by being a very minimalist surgeon and by that I mean do little, if you see what I mean. I don't mean do keyhole surgery, do little, and that would be reflected if you did a longer term follow-up, but that's not the way things are and all of it I find desperately worrying. The implication that there have been a large number of doctors who've not been doing their best or who are substandard is not my impression. It's not what I've seen, now admittedly in neurosurgery you do see a very restricted field, but I don't think I saw in the time that I was in neurosurgery a whole load of bad neurosurgeons. I saw people who were desperately trying to deal with a very difficult situation with the best that they had. I would say that I think the neurosurgical units in many parts of the country have been ill supported. We had to fight for loads of equipment from the word go. Even in the good days there was no rush to give us things like scanners, people weren't keen to provide in theatre many of the equipment pieces that were obviously good in what they would allow you to do, things like ultrasonic dissectors, and for years we were raising money by charity to buy essential equipment. I never see anybody commenting about the actual equipment in hospitals or the paramedical services which all impact on outcome and why don't they comment? I strongly suspect because it's too much to take on board and the results would be frightening because it would be so expensive, wouldn't it. So, 'Let's batter the doctors' seems to be the current view. I must say during latter years I've felt support for doctors has fallen away and away and they've been niggled at by the administration, by patients, even by the law and to my mind it's all going in the wrong direction. And to somebody that's interested in research I think it's making people very, very cautious about going into new avenues of treatment and that has to be the ultimate bad thing. How do you introduce a new treatment now? You can't prove that it's going to be something wonderful and revolutionary until you've actually gone ahead and tried it. I think it's desperately sad. Just take something like hydrocephalus, the current research is beginning to point towards possibilities that the cerebrospinal fluid and its contents might be having a downstream effect. Something that is new and coming in with a lot better understanding of how the brain and CSF systems and so on develop. We might want to start trying to use revolutionary techniques to instil various things into the CSF. How are we going to do it? What we're being told is that you should put in shunts because that is the standard treatment; are we actually going to fossilise medicine at this point? I think it's desperately worrying and sad and I think from all aspects we are being hedged around and not supported, very sad.

"What advice can I give to young people contemplating a career in medicine? I think it's terribly difficult for the reasons that we were saying earlier about the changes in the Health Service because it is no longer what

I would describe as a doctor-friendly career. I actually don't think the opportunities are the same as they were. I think that somebody who is very ambitious is going to find it quite hard now if they have a pioneering spirit because of the legislation that has come in, because of the suspicion, because of the worries too that you might be sued and that your career might come to a sudden end. Look at the number of people who have been suspended and so on. I get shocks when I read some of the medical newspapers and realise just how vulnerable we've all become, but the problem is that if I was now contemplating going into medicine and knew what I know now I wouldn't know what else to do. You know that's the awful thing. I think if somebody is absolutely convinced and is sincere in wanting to do medicine I would support them all the way and I would also hope that they might be able to change the system, that they wouldn't be prepared to put up with some of the legislation which I think now is contrary to anything that we believe in and is against medical practice to be frank, it's supposed to be supporting medicine, but I think it's damaging medicine and I hope that they would see it and fight it. I still feel guilty that my generation didn't fight the changes when they came in. I think we were all slightly complacent and we thought that we were untouchable; maybe that's what made us so vulnerable, isn't it? But I hope the younger generation coming in will perhaps look and pick out what was the best in what I think were the best times and perhaps try and learn from that and bring some of them in again and not be so accepting in a way that we were, I was. I wouldn't stop anybody doing medicine who felt that's what they wanted to do. I don't think there's anything else that would have been right for me. I would have come to the end of my lifetime I think and regretted it terribly. I remember being fascinated by physics when I was, I guess, doing A-levels, but I knew I couldn't do physics, I couldn't have spent a life time doing it, not to make a career of… I couldn't have spent a lifetime in research either. I would have been too frightened that at the end of a lifetime of research I'd actually contributed only perhaps a few very small bricks in a huge big wall and that it really contributed nothing. However, when I look back on medicine, I'm still enormously proud of so many of my patients who I think have done things because they were treated and I wouldn't have missed that. I think the greatest thing of all is to see patients come along with their children and think they might not have been here, you know, so I don't think anything could have compensated for that. No, I would support people who wanted to do medicine provided they were convinced. It's awfully difficult, when I look back I can still remember some of the feelings when I finally decided nothing was going to put me off medicine and I'd say it looked a bit like a Hollywood view of medicine and the reality was totally different. I think it was both more shocking and more challenging. Nothing prepares you really for some of the awful things that happen, but nor can it prepare you for the real highs. I don't think anything has given me such a high as a really difficult operation and coming out and the patient waking up and saying, 'Thank you Doctor,' you know you can't experience anything better than that. (They don't always say thank you.)"

MISS CAROLINE DOIG
Paediatric Surgeon

Caroline qualified in 1962 at St Andrews University. Her home town was Forfar, in Scotland. She attended a state school, Forfar Academy. It was her own decision to study medicine and she applied without discussing it with anyone else either at home or at school.

"At the time I chose my medical school there was no UCCA and St Andrews was nearest home and therefore I chose that. I actually won a bursary to the Dundee part of St. Andrews University and therefore went to Dundee. For the first three years I travelled from home, then after that stayed in residence. There was only one doctor in the family, my uncle, but as a very small child aged about three or four I gave my dolls measles and also blood 'confusions.' He also made me a toy stethoscope. So from a very early age I wanted to do medicine.

"In the final year of medicine at Dundee I decided I wanted to do surgery, but then of course had problems since at that particular time there were very few women in surgery and certainly no women in my own hospitals in the area. I was actively discouraged to do this but continued, being a somewhat determined being. I then eventually found that senior jobs, i.e. SRs etc were unlikely in general surgery and moved laterally into paediatric surgery. People suggested that I would get married and therefore not be interested in continuing surgery and I asked if that was necessarily so. I was working in Darlington in general surgery as an SHO when I began to realise that general surgery for a woman was going to be exceedingly difficult. My cousin at that point was working in paediatrics in 'Sick Kids' in Glasgow and it was through him that I got a job as an SHO in paediatric surgery there, found I liked it and continued on in that speciality. I had started some research when I was in Dundee and having finished my paediatric surgical SHO job I decided that as a woman wanting to do surgery I needed two fellowships and also a thesis, so returned to my home university with Donald Douglas and did research into wound infection and nasal carriage and dissemination of bacteria in theatres for which I got a ChM. This was a useful research, it was a year in the bacteriology lab as well as on the ward. It was useful in the fact that of course wound infection continues to be a problem and I have a whole series of yet to be collated forms from all neonates in St Mary's during my 20, almost 25 years in Manchester so that my interest in wound infection continued.

"After acquiring the Mastership in Surgery and the Edinburgh Fellowship I applied for a general surgical registrar post in Durham. That interview was quite interesting because there were about forty applicants and about ten of us were interviewed. They took a very long time to make the decision when I got the post. I later learned that they had never had a female surgical registrar in Durham before and although my CV was the best they were exceedingly worried about appointing a female surgeon. Interestingly enough the following two people in my post were women. And then at the end of two years there, having got my English Fellowship, I had no job and returned back to Dundee to do a paediatric locum post before getting the senior registrar post in Great Ormond Street.

"Re getting my consultant job in Manchester, I was working as a senior registrar in Great Ormond Street, being there for five years. I applied for the post in Manchester and was given by my professor a good reference, but also he wished me the worst of British luck because he wished me to get a consultant job in London which I am eternally grateful I didn't get. Even before I was appointed consultant in Manchester I did teaching in Great Ormond Street and some clinical research. I thoroughly enjoyed teaching both undergraduates and postgraduates in Manchester and feel probably I was quite good at it perhaps as a hereditary thing since Mother was a good teacher and also enjoyed teaching. It is one of the ways I hope I have helped to influence people.

"Concerning the question of gender discrimination, certainly when I applied for Medical School in St Andrews/Dundee I did not feel any discrimination and a third of our year were at that point women. Nor were there any problems with house jobs as both of mine were in our local teaching hospitals, in fact my surgical job being in the Surgical Professorial Unit. However, once I went further into surgery there was quite definite discrimination although I did actually get the posts, but one was being actively discouraged. However, once I got into paediatric surgery there was absolutely no discrimination against me being a woman at all, but as a young speciality starting just immediately after the war there were always women consultants in it and at the moment something like 19%-20% are women – probably better, for example than paediatric surgery in the States where there are less women than in Britain.

"Two interesting stories. When I decided I wanted to do paediatric surgery, having done an SHO post and liked it, I then went back to my home university and into the Surgical Professorial Unit again to do my research. I then of course was wanting to do general surgery, which I continued in the North of England. Once I wanted to do paediatric surgery I didn't know how to go about it. One of the consultant surgeons who had actively discouraged me early on, then helped me a great deal, arranging for me to meet the professor of paediatric surgery in Great Ormond Street. He gave me advice as to what I should do re getting various qualifications and told me not to be discouraged. I was at that point doing a general surgical job in Durham and felt that if I couldn't proceed in either general surgery or paediatric surgery I would end up doing pathology. He told me not to do this. Some three or four months later there was a post in Great Ormond Street for which I applied and was interviewed (I thought probably because of his influence), I certainly didn't expect to get the post which I did. Also Willie Walker who was a surgeon in Dundee who had helped me and Andrew Wilkinson were prime movers in putting me up for being on the Council of the Royal College of Surgeons of Edinburgh, so throughout my career both of them helped, plus Sir Donald Douglas who was the professor of surgery in Dundee. Interestingly enough both Donald Douglas and Andrew Wilkinson, the professor in paediatric surgery, were ex-presidents of the Royal College of Surgeons of Edinburgh. When I wrote to Andrew Wilkinson before I got the post I pointed out that I now had my English as well as my Edinburgh Fellowship and Mastership he wrote back and said that was excellent, but that he hoped in the future two Fellowships would not be necessary and signed himself Andrew W. Wilkinson ChM,FRCSE,FRCS exactly the same initials as I have. I kept the letter and showed him many years later.

"The other story is to do with paediatric surgery, as an SHO in paediatric surgery I was in Glasgow and working in 'Sick Kids' at a point when it started to fall down. Therefore we were split all over the city and I ended up in Stobhill, an adult hospital, working for a paediatric surgeon for whom I had not worked before called Wallace Dennison. One evening when we were operating he asked why I wanted to do paediatric surgery and I informed him what I wanted to do, the fact that I was going to do research back in Dundee and he suggested that once I got a Thesis and a Mastership then I should come back and he would help me. I don't think he expected me to do it and three years later when I asked him for a reference and told him that I now had my Mastership he of course gave me a very good reference. He used to dine out on the fact that, 'She went off and bloody well did what I told her to do.'

"The personal achievement that pleased me most was being the first woman ever to be on the council of the Royal College of Surgeons of Edinburgh after its inception four hundred years ago. There are now three other woman on the council. I am not however the first woman on a surgical council as Phyllis George was the first one in London."

Caroline has been extremely happy and fulfilled in her career and has never married.

"Although I say I haven't got any great disappointment in my career I am disappointed that I haven't had any children of my own and certainly that was the one and only thing that disappointed my mother."

Caroline and her mother had a close relationship and lived together until her mother's death not long ago. Sadly her father was killed in the Second World War when Caroline was just a little girl. In recent years she finished the dolls' house which he was making for her, thus discovering a fascinating hobby. She has made and furnished several more dolls' houses, constructing miniature household items with great skill and ingenuity.

Caroline believes the NHS is going downhill at the present time but would not discourage young people from choosing medicine as a career provided they are sure that is what they want to do. She considers that women's contribution to medicine should be the same as that of men.

DR. MARY ANDERSON
General Practitioner and Deputy Police Surgeon

I qualified in 1966. I did my preclinical in Oxford and clinical studies at St. Mary's Hospital in London. These were my first choices. I tended to go to places where I knew somebody else who was going. I took no notice of my own GP at home who said Leeds was very good, nor my father's cousin Mildred Creak who said Newcastle would be best.

There were no doctors in my immediate family. Both my parents were musicians. It was very much my own decision to study medicine. I had decided by the age of four that I wanted to be a doctor. I really wanted to be a surgeon, but eczema of the hands was to make that impossible. The situation was complicated by the fact that I also wanted to be a violinist, although my father told me I would never be good enough.

At school (Kendal High School) I kept trying to decide, changing from science to arts subjects and back again. Everyone encouraged me. I got help with extra Latin – an entrance requirement for Oxford at the time. Then my mother died. This was the worst time of my life. My father advised me that perhaps to be a science teacher would be my best bet as it would give me more time to play the violin. By now I had got into the National Youth Orchestra and loved it. My father thought combining medicine and music would be impossible. Perhaps he was right.

I went to St Hilda's College, Oxford, to read chemistry. I soon found chemistry was a big mistake and managed to switch to medicine after all, thanks to the kindness of my tutors and the generosity of my local authority and the Nuffield Foundation who extended my grant. I had a marvellous time in Oxford including heaps of music. I also enjoyed the clinical training in London, and more music. I skimped a bit on ENT in order to get my Violin Teachers Diploma (LRAM).

After qualifying I got my first four jobs easily, but after that it became more difficult. Perhaps because I made some unsuitable applications. I did not have the MRCP, and I applied for various jobs without finding out in advance what they were looking for or what the department was like and so on. Not surprisingly I was unsuccessful. I also became rather depressed, tired and isolated.

Then near the end of one of my hospital jobs I found myself looking after a patient who had returned from relief work in Biafra. He told me something about it. As soon as I could I contacted Save the Children Fund and joined one of their teams for eight months working for the Red Cross in Nigeria.

After the end of the Nigerian Civil War I returned to London. What to do next? I got a part time job in general practice and had more violin lessons. Then I went to Manchester to audition for the Hallé Orchestra, and by a miracle got in. So I gave up medicine completely for nearly five years.

Then I went back to full-time medicine via a job in occupational medicine. Then Paul Miller and I got married. We had known each other since Oxford. We lived in Houston, Texas for 18 months; Paul to do research and me to work in community medicine. I was supposed to set up student electives in local industries. This was difficult because there was some secrecy about occupational hazards; particularly about the clusters of brain tumour cases in communities near petrochemicals in 'Gasoline Alley.' Music helped me. The local classical music radio station KLEF announced which amateur orchestras needed violinists, and where to go to join. That opened other doors – invitations to play chamber music etc. We found Americans very hospitable.

When we returned to England we wanted to start a family. I thought we might not be able to have any children. When none arrived we applied to adopt. Our first two came to us in 1981, when Nick was three and three-quarters and Jackie (his half sister) was 13 months old. Then followed our 'home grown' two. With hindsight it might have been easier to have had our children sooner; but then they wouldn't have been the same people, would they.

I didn't take much time off – perhaps thirteen weeks each time. Coping with family and work was difficult and tiring, particularly for us being older. But this was partly offset by having accumulated more resources. Child care was complicated and expensive. We relied mainly on a series of nannies and au pairs plus some help from friends.

I have worked limited hours ever since, mainly in general practice. I eventually became a partner in the practice where I am now. I never did a trainee year, but got approved by a 'certificate of equivalent experience.' I have since done a stint in hospital again to get on the obstetric list. I have so far avoided being caught up in committee work for the latest NHS reorganisation – Primary Care Groups or Primary Care Trusts. There are quite enough meetings at work already. But in addition to being a GP I am now a Deputy Police Surgeon on the rota for the St Mary's Sexual Assault

Referral Centre. This career path has been a total muddle, the result of chance and impulse. I have enjoyed all these zigzags, but looking back, I wonder if it has just been a case of Attention Deficit Hyperactivity Disorder. What might have been achieved if I'd been single-minded?

I am most grateful to my husband and family for all their understanding and support. They must have suffered from neglect, but still seem to be thriving. None of the children want to do medicine. They don't want to live like us. They think we make work. They say things like 'Stop this project now.' and 'Get a life.'

My principal outside interests are the family, reading, walking and music.

The greatest professional challenge has been combining medicine, music and family. What professional achievement has pleased me most? Well, I got a kick out of passing the MRCGP exam this year, partly to prove to myself that I could, and partly for something to put in my 'Portfolio' towards Revalidation.

But the hardest thing has been keeping going; not giving up; surviving an action against me for alleged negligence in 1968 – over a child's death that occurred two weeks into my surgical house job. The case was settled out of court. The whole experience was terrible in every way, and is always with me. I believe that nowadays there is more emotional and practical support.

The NHS? I think NHS is a marvellous idea and has treated me and my family wonderfully well as patients. Unfortunately it seems under threat just now. I can't remember health care before the NHS, but I do remember a lot of children in our village school suddenly getting spectacles and going to the dentist.

The greatest challenge for medicine? Stop smoking! Globally the old problems are still there – poverty, poor water, malaria, war, and famine. In this country the challenge is people need to be more self-reliant. We have over-medicalised everyone and everything. Nobody dares to feel normal any more. A challenge for our society will be helping people to trust their common sense over minor ailments, and trust their own self-healing. Another challenge for doctors is going to be how to cope with information overload. Patients are suffering from this too, because although medical knowledge is exciting and fascinating, more information does not always make you feel well or confident.

Contribution of women doctors? – potentially as valuable as any. But many women doctors are too busy and have to rush home after work so they're not around to be role models. Many women need support and encouragement to put themselves forward and to get as good a deal as their male counterparts; fair pay and conditions, and equality of opportunity. This is how MWF has helped me; with role models and advice.

Advice to young people contemplating medicine, based on what I would do differently if I had another chance. Ask for help and information as often as you need it. Don't get to feel isolated. Look after yourself, your hobbies and your friends. Do what makes you happy.

DR. HILARY HARRIS
General Practitioner

Hilary qualified at Liverpool University Medical School in 1967. Liverpool was not her first choice.

"I would have much preferred to go to London or Oxford or Cambridge, but at that time there were really no other pupils at the school who'd ever been to London or very rarely to medical school at all, so that was a bit discouraging and I think it was easier to get in, certainly to Oxbridge, if there had been other people before you or perhaps if you were cleverer than I am or was. I felt a bit persuaded to go to Liverpool because it was much cheaper to go to Liverpool, and my parents would have had some difficulty at the time in trying to support me away from home, but subsequently I very much wished I had gone away from home because it was very difficult living at home initially and being at medical school. I think that was probably one of the reasons why I married early."

Although there were no other doctors in the family, Hilary's parents encouraged her ambition to read medicine. However her school, which was in the state system, was not so supportive.

"There was quite a lot of discouragement about applying for medicine from school. Their range of activities didn't seem to go much beyond nursing and it was very much, 'Well, apply if you want to but we really don't think you'll get in,' which wasn't at all encouraging at the time. I have to say that I felt that this was very much the case even at Altrincham Grammar School in the 80's when my daughter was applying for medical school, this again wasn't encouraging.

"I haven't had an awful lot of difficulty in getting posts after qualification except on one occasion when I felt there was a fair amount of discrimination, and that was actually obtaining my second house job. I did my first house job away from Liverpool in the South of England, in Dartford, and when I came to get the house surgical post which I thought would just be automatic I was told all the posts in Dartford were already allocated to London Medical School. This was very miffing indeed and I then had to move to High Wycombe in Buckinghamshire because at the time I needed accommodation for myself and my daughter and a nanny, as my husband was in the forces and away from home, so that was quite a challenging time, quite difficult and difficult anyway to obtain any accommodation for children at that point.

"It wasn't a long-held preference to be a GP at all. I would much have preferred to have been a paediatrician and always would, and still would have liked to have been a paediatrician but it was really impossible because I had a daughter already and it was very difficult to do any sort of long-term residential work with a small child so I somewhat drifted into general practice. I did do a year of radiology and got first part of DMRD and then really found that this was something I didn't like doing at all, I really missed the patient contact. What I'd been hoping to do and why I chose radiology was really to go up the consultant path quite quickly, which I think I probably would have done had I stayed in it, but I don't think it was a career option that I would have found very fulfilling.

"Outside interests. Well, I had to think about this one, which means that I haven't got very many. I've got lots of ones on the horizon but none that I have any time to do properly and that makes me worry a bit about retirement and whether you really can have a retirement on which you haven't really built at all for the future, so my interests really are family, I've got an enormous family and they keep me pretty occupied, and my other interest is ballet which I go to an awful lot and which I would love to develop more interest in.

"I married twice. First not a success but I'm quite sure that was the combination of trying to combine being a medical student, qualifying and starting on a career with marriage, a very bad combination and one that I think my daughter considered very carefully when she was choosing medicine. Second one I think has been a lot more satisfactory but we were both very established in our individual careers at that point. Both my husbands are doctors. My only daughter was born two years before qualification, not after qualification, this brought its own problems and she was unplanned, although definitely not unwanted, and we were married for some time before she arrived. I definitely would have changed the timing of my family and had them post qualification and post a bit of postgraduate work as well. I had virtually no time off at all, being a medical student, although I was urged to have a year off by the Dean of the Medical School but didn't take that option, probably should have done. On my second marriage I took on two children, my husband's by his first marriage. His children are adopted children, his first wife had died. I worked part-time for some considerable time after we had married because obviously bringing a family together who had had some difficulties individually was quite challenging. I think that's worked pretty well although I was a bit concerned that my son said that he definitely wouldn't want to marry a woman doctor himself, which probably speaks a lot. I have been very fortunate in terms of childcare all along in that my mother was very, very helpful indeed. She was a career person herself, a headmistress, but she somehow managed to combine looking after one and then three children of mine and allowing me to do an awful lot of things that wouldn't have been possible without her and my father's input, that was an enormous help. I don't think that could ever have been substituted by paying. My biological daughter has followed me into medicine and is a consultant dermatologist and seems to be very happy.

"I think my greatest challenge has been trying to combine a real outside interest in medicine with being a GP. I think that's continuing to be very difficult. My interest is in genetics so it leads me on to my greatest achievement which I think is being appointed to the Human Genetics Commission, but trying to combine that is very difficult and I really now need to go very part-time because it's impossible to do all the genetics work. My difficulty is that I took on the general practice, it's mine, I have a partner but I own the building and therefore there's an awful lot of investment, I don't mean financial investment, in it. It is also a very happy place to work. I enjoy it a great deal but I really have to give up an awful lot of that if I'm going to do the genetics work in the future. My disappointment… not so much a disappointment, my only real difficulty in my career was one difficulty with a partnership which was extremely troublesome and which I left, and made me for a time feel that perhaps medicine, or perhaps general practice, was not the career for me and made me very determined to at some point set up my own practice and choose my own partner and direct myself, which I think altogether has been very satisfactory and successful. I've had two partners and they've both been extremely good. The first one left because her husband moved area.

"I'm pretty pessimistic about the NHS at the moment despite all this new money that is going to be thrown at us. I don't like primary care groups, now ours is a primary care trust, if I'd wanted to be a groupie I'd have done something else. I'm not happy about the way things are going at all and the degree of control that the trust is going to exert upon us and that this doesn't allow us to have the autonomy that we had before. I know we're in the very early stages of trusts but I'm not very happy about it. I think for medicine in the future trying to combine the enormous technological advances that are happening in all aspects of medicine with delivering a caring and empathy-led service is going to be very difficult and I don't know where the balance is going to come down. I think the continuing interference of Government is very challenging and I don't think that's going to go away at all.

"I am very positive about women in medicine. I think they make an enormous contribution and will continue to do so and I think the move to more part-time medicine and also to salaried medicine is probably a great plus for women doctors, but I think there will always be difficulties because childcare will ultimately devolve to women, inevitably.

"I have been influenced by the MWF. I went to one conference abroad where I represented the MWF and found that very interesting and I was very glad to have been asked. I read the magazine. I don't take a great deal of active part because of my other outside interests, I'd like to but there just isn't time. I definitely would promote medicine as a career for young people, I've always felt this because I think it offers such a lot of opportunities, such a lot of different career paths. I think you can even be in medicine somebody who actually doesn't like people all that much, but there will be a role for you if you find that out by the time you've qualified, and there are many, many options. So I think there's a place for everybody in medicine and there are very few careers that offer all of that."

PROFESSOR DIAN DONNAI
Geneticist

Dian qualified in 1968 at St Mary's Hospital Medical School, University of London. She came from a non-medical family and was grateful that her state school vigorously encouraged her to do medicine.

"I was born in Shropshire, rural Shropshire in a small town which I think at that time had about two or three thousand people in it, called Whitchurch. It was about 20 miles from Chester and 20 miles from Shrewsbury and you really only went out of Whitchurch to buy a new winter coat or to see Father Christmas. It was really quite an isolated little country town, but it was a market town so there was sufficient there to mean you didn't need to go out and I think it was quite a sort of inward-looking place.

"I was born at the end of the war. I was a twin and I was born in the back bedroom at home, my mother previously having had a baby that was premature and was a neonatal death. We were delivered by the local GP and the midwife and the GP was always my mother's hero. He was called Dr Clayton, Dr Edgar Clayton and he was an FRCS and he smoked and he drank and he had diabetes but he was sort of god-like in my parents' eyes. I was born weighing 4lbs, I was the first one out; I was born just before midnight and my twin brother was born just after midnight. So I grew up and I've always thought this may be one of the reasons I went into genetics, I think there are more people who are twins in genetics and more people who are left-handers in genetics and that might be because they see themselves as just that little bit different. I don't know, it's an unproven theory.

"I went to the little Whitchurch infant school and then transferred to the Whitchurch junior school and I suppose I might have been reasonably able at that time because I was put straight into the second year in the junior school, so ended up doing my eleven-plus a year early and went to what was called Whitchurch Girls' High School with in total I think about 120 girls in the school, a very small school. I think we did biology for O-level, there was no science, they didn't have chemistry or physics.

"When I was about thirteen I went into hospital because I had a lump on my arm which was a bony exostosis and I went to Oswestry Orthopaedic Hospital. I was quite fascinated by the whole hospital environment and I think it was probably that that made me think about going into medicine, but I didn't think about going into medicine straight away, I thought about physiotherapy and sent off for all the bits of paper about physiotherapy and it was my headmistress who suggested medicine to me. My family were poor, my dad was a labourer and my mum didn't work, she'd had another baby by then so there were the three of us altogether and I remember my dad earning twenty pounds per week and handing it over to my mum and her putting piles for the milk and for the meat and everything. Neither of them had had any secondary education and my mum had no parents because her mum died of a thrombosis after she was born and she was brought up by her sisters, and my dad's dad died when he was about four. So we were quite a poor family, but respectable because in fact my mum had inherited a very small inheritance and they did own their own house, a small semi-detached house in Whitchurch but the thought of professional education was something that wasn't within their experience or indeed mine. But this rather exceptional headmistress called Molly Dennis, who actually went on to be the headmistress of the North London Collegiate School for Girls, had obviously spotted me as having some potential and talked to me about my career when I was doing O-levels and I said about physiotherapy and she said, "Why don't you think about medicine?'

"So I remember going home and telling my parents about it that night and they were horrified. This was only fairly soon after the introduction of the health service and so they said there was no way I could do medicine because they couldn't afford to send me to university and they couldn't afford to buy me a practice, because that was their view of what medicine particularly involved. But the headmistress had obviously taken me on as a sort of cause. So after I'd done O-levels (and I failed Latin, that's the only exam that I ever failed, I failed Latin and had to do it again), I could do at my school botany and zoology which I had to do at A-level but for physics and chemistry I had to have special arrangements to go to the boys' school. That was only a little bigger, probably about two hundred boys, and I used to have to ride up on my bike for every chemistry and physics lesson and it used to add another hour and half to my day going back and forth. They had to make special arrangements for me to use the headmaster's toilet and one of the teachers, the chemistry teacher, said he'd never taught a girl in his life and he wasn't going to start, and so he called me Charlie from the day I went there. Anyway I had to do chemistry and physics from scratch joining the boys in the sixth form. I did O-level chemistry and physics after the first year and A-level after the second year.

"At that time I then applied to do medicine. I sent off for lots of forms from various places: Birmingham, Manchester, and London but I rather fancied going to London. Nobody ever suggested Oxford or Cambridge or anything like that so I fancied London and I sent to, I remember, Guy's and St Thomas's and Bart's and maybe the Middlesex and St Mary's, Paddington and on most of the forms one of the questions was, 'Is your father a member of the medical, legal or clerical profession?' And I looked at that and thought I would never get in to any of these places and so I didn't apply for those. But the one that didn't ask that was St. Mary's in Paddington which was where I decided, okay, I was going to go. So I had to go off for an interview and I remember having to walk to the station and getting a train to Crewe and then getting a train to Paddington, but at least the trains ran on time in those days and I could do it there and back in a day. I can still remember walking into the big boardroom there and being interviewed by a guy who I think was a dermatologist, now I think about it. Anyway I must have sounded terribly naïve but obviously they must have thought I had something about me and so they accepted me subject to A-levels. Well, I worked harder then than I've ever worked in my whole life, I think, doing these four A-levels, two from scratch, I really worked hard and eventually did A-levels and got them. I don't think we had grades in those days, thank goodness, because I don't imagine my chemistry or physics would have been very good.

"Then I got into medical school but I was too young, I was still only seventeen so I had to wait around for a year and my parents were terrified that I might fall off the academic ladder and that if I went out to work I would never get back into the habit of studying and there were no real options. So I had to go back to school for a year, I did English A-level for the last year there and eventually then left this little country school. In the final year, because I'd got my A-levels this headmistress had encouraged me or I think she even sent the forms in for me to apply for the entrance scholarships to St. Mary's. I had to go for another interview up to London and eventually I was given the major entrance scholarship for St. Mary's. That was a hundred pounds a year and since the grant for each term was only a hundred pounds anyway, it was like another term's grant. I obviously got a full grant. I have to say unlike my kids at university I was never in debt and I think I even saved some money because of this scholarship thing, so it was quite extraordinary.

"Anyway there I was, I'd left this little country town, it was horrible trying to find accommodation and I stayed with a friend of mine from school who'd gone to music college in London for the first term, she and I shared a room, and then eventually I got into the hall of residence and things were okay. So I started at St. Mary's, Paddington. There were seventy people in the year and I think there were probably about fourteen women, fourteen out of seventy, but they were a good group and I soon got to know people and we were all from very different backgrounds. The friend that I'm still in touch with from there was rather smart, her brothers had gone to Eton and she'd gone away to boarding school but we got on well and still get on very well, so in fact by that time the backgrounds didn't matter at all.

"I think I was just like any other student, I didn't particularly like the first eighteen months which was just the anatomy and physiology and biochemistry. We used to do quite a lot of interesting things as well, the students at St. Mary's used to be film extras so I've actually had tiny bit extra parts in quite a lot of movies that are still shown like 'Doctor in Clover' and my husband was in 'Those Magnificent Men in their Flying Machines,' I was in 'Arabesque' with Gregory Peck and Sophia Loren. So these were things we used to do to earn a bit of extra money which was quite amusing, but after the first eighteen months we started on the wards; that's when I felt I really was doing what I wanted to do. I really enjoyed the exposure to clinical medicine, it's all obviously lost a bit in the mists of time but the attachments that I really liked were the ones where you actually got to do something or people talked to you. The ones that I liked best were the paediatric options. There was a terrific professor of paediatrics called Tom Oppé and I'm still in touch with him and regard him really as my mentor in medicine. He was really good at looking at the whole family, St Mary's had a home care team way before there was any such thing as community paediatrics and he also had a neonatal unit and we used to talk about the families and how they felt. So this really brought the whole business alive to me and this is probably what started my interest in paediatric aspects.

"I also enjoyed obstetrics, the fact that we were privileged to have to be able to deliver babies and I think I quite liked the A&E attachments too because you got to do a few things, those were the subjects that really stand out, particularly the paediatrics because I really liked the whole environment. So I decided before I finished as a student that I probably wanted to follow a paediatric path. The thing I definitely did not like was surgery and the reason for this was partly because one was treated with such contempt by the actual surgeons that were around. I remember male student colleagues of mine, the more these surgeons shouted the more they were impressed by them. There was one surgeon who used to throw things on the floor and this particularly impressed male colleagues of mine. I just thought this was terrible and there is one incident that I really would like to record, I just hope that people would never do these things again. In this incident, I can still remember the ward, I was on a ward round with a surgeon and there was a whole group of students, probably about fifteen on a big Nightingale ward and I can still remember exactly where on the ward this bed was. There was a woman in it who had previously had a mastectomy for breast cancer and she had got a recurrent tumour of the breast. This surgeon, because we couldn't all get round the bed, didn't put the curtains round, he opened her nightdress and he drew on her chest with a felt tip pen to show where he was going to do the incision and I just remember being so horrified, thinking this could be my mother sitting in that bed. I think I remember going up to talk to this woman after the students moved away and holding her hand under the bedclothes and getting shouted at for lagging behind, but that was the most horrific memory of my time as a medical student and I just think it's worth recording that those things were still happening in the late sixties, this would be about 1967. I thought I'd just mention that.

"Anyway I chose not to go into surgery, not surprisingly, and decided to do paediatrics. At St. Mary's you could do paediatrics as a pre-registration house-job, and Prof Oppé, I think, was famous for actually choosing women to do this particular job. There were some quite distinguished women who preceded me in this job. We used to have to work every other night on call and when we were on call we used to have to cover the ENT ward, and in addition to every other night on call we had to do one night in casualty a week in Paddington casualty which was heavy duty, you were the first line there. I forgot to say in all of this, of course, that while I was a medical student I had met my husband-to-be, who's still my husband, he's also a medic, he was at St. Mary's although he'd been to Cambridge first and was a couple of years ahead of me and actually we married just about three or four months before I did 2nd MB. We used to qualify on the Conjoint exams too so that you could do some paid locums in your last few months, so I did that in December, I think, and then we got married in January and I got my MB in April or May and started to work in the

August. So we got married, I think we rented a flat, but since he was working two nights out of three and I was working every other night, we only used to see each other about one night out of six, so that meant we didn't really live together until we'd been married four or five years.

"I did my pre-registration job in paediatrics which of course I really enjoyed and I then went and did a house surgery job in Ealing and I enjoyed that too. Then I think I went back to St. Mary's and did an obstetric job because I really felt that if I was going to do paediatrics, and I was really rather interested more in the neonatal side of things, that I needed some obstetrics, so I did a six month obstetric job. But I have to say when I was doing the obstetric job I was actually more interested in the babies that came out, I remember helping at a caesarean section and realising a baby needed resuscitation and so excusing myself from the surgery and taking over the baby bit. Then after I'd done that I decided that I needed to concentrate on getting my Membership so my fourth job was in general medicine because you couldn't do paediatric Membership then, you could do a paediatric clinical but you had to do a general medicine viva and exam. So I went to West Middlesex Hospital where I took a job on the gastroenterology unit with two people, Dr Stewart and Dr Coghill, who made a big impression on me, because I was really impressed by the way he spoke to patients. He was a terrific guy and he was the most civilised person to patients and I remember learning a lot from him on how to give families bad news.

"So I did that and I must have done Part One at the end of that, then I was asked by someone who had also worked for Professor Oppé in paediatrics to go and work with her. She had just been appointed as consultant at the hospital which was just about to open called Northwick Park Hospital, she was a paediatrician called Betty Priestley. She asked me to go and work with her as her SHO, that was the only member of junior staff she had, so I took that post and was there at the beginning of that hospital. It had a research focus because it was partly funded by research funding, there were research wards and there were service wards and during the time I was there I did Part Two Membership and passed it, thank goodness.

"When I finished that my plans were that I would apply and try and get a job at Great Ormond Street which I'd got everything together to try and do, then my husband got a job in Sheffield so I had to forget Great Ormond Street and think in terms of Sheffield. I applied for a registrar job that was being advertised in Sheffield and went and was interviewed for this job and they spent the whole of the interview asking me what my reproductive plans were, the whole time, I remember nothing much else and I didn't get the job, but interestingly enough one of the people on the committee was Professor Victor Dubowitz who was actually a senior lecturer at the time. It must have been twenty-odd years later, I know him from overlap in the genetics field, that he said to me he'd always remembered that interview and how awful it was and how embarrassed he felt because he felt all the questioning was totally inappropriate, but actually I said to him they'd probably done me a favour because it meant I didn't get the job, I didn't get funnelled into paediatrics and when the opportunity came up to do genetics it was an option for me so actually it was probably a good turn. So, I spent the two years we were in Sheffield working half-time in the casualty department with Cynthia Illingworth as an accident and emergency registrar and half-time in a general practice with a single-handed GP, I was a half-time assistant to him and again I learnt a huge amount from that. And I used to moonlight on the special care unit at night doing locum cover in Sheffield.

"Anyway eventually my husband's career then took him to Manchester and so I ended up in Manchester in 1972. At that time we had been hoping to have a family but it had taken a long time. I'd had a miscarriage and then I still wasn't becoming pregnant and so that was really my priority when we got to Manchester. I was given a bit of Clomid, that was the thing they were giving at the time. Anyway eventually I did become pregnant, it wasn't a straightforward pregnancy but happily it resulted in the birth of my daughter in 1974. By this time I hadn't worked for a year and a bit, although I did some GP locums and then I think my son Tom was born within about 14 months so we'd obviously got the recipe right at this stage.

"So I had two children very quickly but was really missing doing medicine, I found it very hard not to be involved because I really loved the hospital environment and I was a bit worried about where my career was likely to go. In fact what happened was my husband was speaking to Dr Rodney Harris who ran the genetics department at St. Mary's and he mentioned that he had got some sessions, clinical assistant sessions and would I be interested in them. I looked into the childcare facilities, luckily at the MRI at the time there was a crèche space, so I took two half sessions a week as a clinical assistant, this was in 1977. As soon as I got into the specialty of genetics which was really very much an emerging specialty at the time, I realised that this was where I was always meant to be, everything I'd done up till then was really an interest. I'd always been interested in paediatrics in children with birth defects of various sorts and I'd been interested in the response of whole families to situations and so this was really just terrific. So I ended up, since I was paying for the crèche for the whole day, working for two whole days even though I was only being paid for two half days and got more and more involved. Because Dr Harris, who subsequently became Professor Harris, had a background in adult medicine, this really gave me a free rein to try and develop the paediatric aspect of genetics and during the course of that year there was an opportunity to develop a job description for a senior registrar. Up to then there were no senior registrars in genetics but two were developed during that year, one in Manchester and one at Northwick Park that was eventually taken by my friend and colleague Robin Winter who is now professor at Great Ormond Street. So he and I were the first senior registrars in genetics in the UK, together with another post in Wales soon afterwards and Ian Young who later became a professor in Nottingham was appointed to that.

"So we were the first three SRs in genetics in the country and really things just developed from there, I developed more of my interest in genetics and made more network connections with other people working in the field, got more and more interested in patterns of birth defects and ended up making national and international connections and really that's what I've been doing ever since. Eventually I got a consultant job, I was appointed as SR in 1978 and then as a consultant late in 1980 so I've been a consultant since then. I have concentrated on developing the paediatric aspect of genetics within the regional genetics service, but also developing aspects of foetal genetics because I felt a lot of babies identified through prenatal diagnosis were not getting the full range of investigations to establish a diagnosis. Similarly with children, people in paediatrics had tended to look at the mortality and morbidity and just put congenital malformations as a sort of wodge at the bottom and implied that that was something that nothing could be done about. So I felt that maybe these families required different sorts of services and that's what I've always been very keen to try and develop. People want to know what the problem is and why it happened and what it means for the child and will it happen again. I think the focus of my work in birth defects has been largely towards answering those sorts of questions and also for those conditions where there haven't been answers, trying to undertake clinical research and then linking with scientific research to try and develop answers in those sorts of fields. So that's been the main focus of my clinical and scientific work. More recently of course you get dragged into committees the older you get, so I've taken on quite a lot of other sorts of responsibilities.

"I was given an honorary chair in 1993/1994 which I was very flattered by and honoured and that's been a great pleasure to me. It was rather sad that I got that about a year after both my parents died at the age of eighty-something within about six weeks of each other, they never did get to know that bit about my career but never mind.

"I've obviously taken on more responsibilities nationally. By 1984 I'd made lots of connections in the United States and started going to dysmorphology meetings in the United States and making connections there and I thought this is something we ought to be doing in Europe as well. So in 1984 I set up the Manchester Birth Defects Conferences and we've had them every two years since 1984. They've been incredibly successful, people fight to get places in these meetings so we really get a lot of people from the US now and Australia and from the rest of Europe. So that's one thing that I'm very pleased we've developed within Manchester.

"The other thing is obviously that a lot of people work within the Regional Genetic Service based in St. Mary's and all of them have made big individual contributions to the development of the speciality and to the department. I've been Clinical Director for about the last five years and we've seen consultant numbers increasing by about four in that period so it is certainly a growing field, but it obviously involves a lot of management and administrative work to try and get these developments in place."

Dian is keen to encourage all members of her staff to take responsibility in their own special area and have a say in the general organisation. Flexibility and family-friendliness are important features of department policy.

When she has time Dian enjoys travelling, going to the gym, reading and bird-watching for relaxation. She is optimistic about the NHS, convinced it is better than the alternative and currently improving, though meeting demand and finding resources remain the greatest challenges. She is sure women doctors can make a huge contribution, bringing a new openness and style to the establishment.

Her advice to young people contemplating a medical career is only to do it if really sure it is what they want. Her own children are not following their parents into medicine.

DR. HELEN LEWIS
Paediatrician

Helen trained at Oxford and the Middlesex Hospital and qualified in 1971. There were other doctors in her family but it was her own idea to study medicine. She was not discouraged in this aspiration either at home or at her school, which was a direct grant school, and was fortunate enough to get into the medical school of her choice. Once qualified she set about realising her ambition of becoming a consultant paediatrician, but there were difficulties along the way.

"I didn't have any difficulties with my pre-registration house posts but after I finished my house jobs and applied for an SHO post I had probably five or six interviews for paediatrics, which was my career of first choice, and although I was short-listed for all of them I wasn't given any offers and was actually asked bluntly at nearly every interview, 'What's the point of training a woman in a hospital career?' because I was married by that stage. I had answers to that, but decided I had better broaden my experience in case I did not become a paediatrician after all. I applied for posts that were easier to obtain at the time. I did a medical SHO post, which was easier, and obstetrics and gynae, and then I had no difficulty in finding a paediatric post after that.

"After I had completed one year as a paediatric SHO and had got my Part 1 MRCP and my DCH I was pregnant but I was encouraged to continue in my career by the consultants I was working for, who were very supportive. They introduced me to another lady who was one of the first doctors on the flexible training scheme and she told me how to go about it. At the time I had to get sponsored by a consultant who thought he could do with a supernumerary registrar. There was no general application scheme. So by personal contact, I was put in touch with Dr Bernard Valman at Northwick Park and he was, and still is, a man who knows how to do things. So he put in all the necessary applications on my behalf and applications for funding and special permission for a supernumerary post which had to go then directly to the Ministry of Health. It was turned down because it was said at the time, which was in 1975, that paediatrics was a specialty which was going to steadily decline because children were so healthy and therefore, as now, they said we're only going to recruit supernumerary doctors in specialties where there will be a good chance of a consultant career. So it was suggested that I retrained in geriatrics and I do still have in my possession, I think, a letter from the Minister of Health at the time to say that.

"When I told Dr Valman he suggested that I write and ask my MP, Margaret Thatcher, who'd just been made Chairman of the Conservative party. We lived in her constituency of North Finchley. I wrote a nice letter to Mrs Thatcher and a few days later, after she received the letter, she made a speech at a major political meeting, I think it might have been the Conservative Annual Party Conference, saying what she was going to do with the health service and how she was going to encourage women to continue in their medical careers and she quoted my case, of a young doctor who had come to a standstill in her career because of administrative problems and had been kept waiting months for a reply. Then by the next post I got a letter from the Ministry of Health. The Minister of Health then was Labour. So my post was approved after a very short time and it was all due to the letter from Mrs Thatcher, which she signed, and I still keep that but it doesn't mean that I supported her for the next twenty-five years. I was part-time registrar at Northwick Park and I was there as a registrar for four years, then I became senior registrar at Northwick Park and then it was easy to transfer to Manchester and I've not had any problems with obtaining posts since then. I was in the right place at the right time. It was pure luck."

Helen got married six months before qualifying. Her husband is a dentist. The first of their four children was planned and arrived when they had been married for three years. Helen took the statutory 18 weeks of maternity leave after each birth. It has not always been easy to fit in home and children with work, but Helen has no regrets about the timing of her family. While always so busy, she has somehow found the energy to keep up other interests such as cycling, swimming, skiing and the theatre.

"In retrospect I don't know how I managed, having four children, except that I had them one at a time. I think it's something you take on more when you are young – what comes at you – for me if I give up and take things more easily then I don't want to go back working harder than I ever did before. So I suppose I coped by just taking on what I had to do. I've always had good support. My mother's always been there in the background. Although she's not provided full-time care, she has always been there in an emergency to help look after the children. I've had residential nannies but I don't think I'd do the same again because we employed inadequately trained nannies, actually, who were too young and I didn't think too deeply about the risks and responsibilities at the time. So nowadays, I think people are more careful. I actually had very good help but didn't think too much about the possible risks of somebody else looking after my children at home. The problem is that paying for good childcare is very expensive. Junior doctors' salaries were not enough at that stage to even financially break even, if you were working and having good domestic support. So I had good but cheap domestic support, relatively, and had to buy a house big enough for the nanny to live in and have some of her own privacy. I only managed to do that because my husband was a consultant by that time, so he could help to support a working wife.

"So having coped with the home and young children it is now financially worthwhile but it was difficult at the time, and I did often think if I didn't get to a consultant post in the future then it would not be a long-term financial proposition for me to continue working at that level. I hear a lot of young women doctors saying they have to let their career work round the childcare arrangements, so there has to be somebody to take the child to nursery or to pick the children up from school, and when I suggest to them that they might have a private arrangement for somebody to come into the home they say, 'Oh we don't want anyone invading our privacy.' One thing that I've learnt is that children (and we) can grow up quite well with a relative stranger in the home and it's a learning experience for all of us, they do become one of the family and you do get to trust people living in your home, even though you might consider it better not to have someone from outside. Now, I don't think I would like to have anybody else in the house, but then I'm used to just having our own privacy and have been for the last few years. One of the things to point out about paying for childcare is it is paid for out of taxed income so it is relatively more expensive."

Helen believes the demands of an ageing and increasingly disabled population will present a huge challenge to medicine in the future, together with the implications of developments in genetics. She is concerned that the NHS is already failing to meet 21st century expectations.

"I have supported the concept of a national health service as the best way of providing good healthcare for all, up until the last year or so. I am now realising, like most other people, that the English system does not provide the best healthcare in the world. In every other sphere the customer can choose what they want to get out of a service and pay accordingly and I feel the public has far too great expectations for the health service and that the services offered will need to be cut down. The demands of the public will have to be adjusted to their priorities and to what some other people could afford to pay for."

Helen considers that women doctors are still undervalued in spite of their abilities.

"Women doctors will have to make a big contribution to British medicine because more than half the medical undergraduates now are women, but as the number of part-time posts has not increased in proportion to the number of women I think that there will be a net loss of doctors to the profession, for some women will choose not to work or to work on a very part-time basis. So I think that it will be relatively easier for men to reach top posts. Therefore, we will continue to be dependent on foreign doctors and on men. So I think men have very good prospects for their careers but women will still be fighting for the same few good posts and for the ability to be able to combine their careers with their families."

Being awarded a DM degree was the professional achievement which has pleased Helen the most. Obtaining recognition of the value of her part-time training has been the hardest professional challenge she has had to meet. Despite all the difficulties, she is glad that one of her daughters is following her into medicine, which she still considers to be a rewarding career. She gives the following advice to girls considering medicine.

"I would advise only to embark on it if you feel strongly committed to medicine and realise that the training will continue for nearly all your young adult life. Exams will continue for all your young adult life. Pay will be less than you will see your friends and colleagues getting, job satisfaction should be good as long as you enjoy what you are doing, but there is no job security in terms of place of work and type of work anymore. I think there is still job security in as much as there will always be work for you to do, but it might not be work of your first choice in the place and time that you want it. So I would advise girls starting in medicine to be aware of all the pitfalls and to be committed, but maintain a fairly open mind as to what specialty you will go into in the end, and be prepared to try your second choice if your first doesn't succeed."

DR. CAROL EWING
Job-sharing Paediatrician and
Associate Dean for Flexible Training, NW Region

There were no other doctors in Carol's family. Her parents were very keen for her to study medicine as this was her wish and she was very supported by her family. She went to St. Andrews and Manchester and qualified in 1978.

"Was I discouraged at school? It was interesting to be at a Northern Ireland grammar school in the late 60's and early 70's because there was a terrific drive to encourage all pupils to make something of their life and to take further education opportunities wherever possible, and sadly this meant there was an exodus of many people aged between 17 and 18 at that time going to colleges outside Northern Ireland, because it coincided with the difficulties Northern Ireland was facing at the time. So we were positively encouraged, but sadly it had an adverse effect for future developments in Northern Ireland as some students had left to go to the mainland.

"Why did I choose St. Andrews University? It was quite an interesting story. My father was appointed as a Registrar in the New University of Ulster in the late 60's and he was given a remit really, of looking at all the universities in England, Wales and Scotland which were built in a new style and so we toured around for a summer holiday and looked at them. We also visited a colleague of his who was the Registrar at St. Andrews University and I fell in love with the town. The fact that it was beside the sea figured highly in my choice of university. I also liked it because it was a Scottish medical school and the first year was accommodating Scottish graduates who came in having done their Higher examinations. I was already up to speed with physics, chemistry and biology and it gave me a chance to go to fine arts lectures and theology lectures and other lectures which were not on the medical course. That was not what was supposed to happen but that's what happened in reality. Coming to Manchester was quite a different challenge, a very different environment but I welcomed it and I thoroughly enjoyed my undergraduate training here, I met my husband and we've been in Manchester ever since."

After qualifying Carol had no difficulties obtaining posts until she came to have children. In deciding on her eventual career, for a time she thought the pathway to becoming a consultant would be too difficult to juggle with family life. She got married four years after qualifying and had her first baby two years later. By that time she was already set on a career in paediatrics.

"In terms of me changing my mind, I was debating whether to follow a career in general practice when I was an SHO. I worked for a year as an SHO at Booth Hall followed by a year in obstetrics and gynaecology which I found incredibly useful but that absolutely focused me back to a paediatric pathway and I then fully plunged into six months of neonatology and was quite focused on a paediatric career after that. I did consider going into community paediatrics but some of the mentors whom I have had in my life, for example Dr Barbara Phillips, Paediatric A&E Consultant, Alder Hey, who has been of immense help to me, strongly encouraged me to keep in acute hospital paediatrics as she felt that I was very suited to that specialty.

"My career pathway was that I worked as a full-time registrar until 1984 by which time I had my MRCP. At that time then I decided that I had no option but to resign from paediatrics, have my baby as I was expecting at that time, and then really look at career options once the baby was born. It was during this time that I went to meet with Dr Ilfra Goldberg who at that time was the Associate Dean with responsibility for flexible training for North West Region and she encouraged me to apply for the PM79(3) scheme." [Part-time training posts were few and far between at that time, and were administered centrally from London under this scheme].

"I will tell you about the interview for the PM79 (3) scheme. I applied for the scheme; it was an interview which took place on an annual basis. The interview took place about ten days after I'd had my second baby son. I actually got over the birth very quickly, but much to the midwife's concern I had to get her agreement to my travelling to London with the baby. Fortunately my mother-in-law who lives in London came up to Manchester and accompanied me down to London and I stayed with her the previous night, which was spent mostly breastfeeding my hungry newborn son. When I arrived at the Health Authority building for the interview they were shocked that I had a newborn baby with me. Fortunately my mother-in-law was able to look after him whilst I was interviewed. Again, I got the distinct impression that the panel thought what was I doing there, as I should be at home with my new baby, until I pointed out to them that actually this was the only opportunity for me to work in this following year. The interview went okay and I returned to Manchester. It was an incredibly difficult journey. What happened was that pylons had come down on the line, so the trains were not coming out of Euston but only out of St. Pancras, so I had to run to St. Pancras from Euston to get the last train to Manchester. It happened to coincide with a football match in Sheffield, so that it was standing room only on the train with hundreds of football supporters who had had rather a lot to drink. I spent my time protected by a large Australian male who was hitchhiking around the U.K. who protected my space with my newborn baby in a Moses basket on the floor, so that I was not knocked over by drunken football hooligans. It was a six-hour journey back to Manchester. Fortunately my baby managed to take a bottle of expressed breast milk, otherwise I don't know how I would have managed and I got back to Manchester at some hour in the early morning.

"After all that, my application was unsuccessful, but afterwards I obtained a research post at Booth Hall with Professor Tim David and that went very well and I eventually acquired my MD out of this work. So there was a nice end to the tale.

"In terms of having a family and timing, I felt that it was time for me to get on and have a family, being thirty when Dan my eldest child was born. There were difficulties which arose when he was ten months old, as my father died suddenly and this contributed to my decision to delay returning to work. I think I was a little bit better with number two and number three, although with the second baby I was carrying out my research work at Booth Hall and I actually worked right up to the birth and was back at work within a week or two, trying to get my research completed. I was continuing with my research actually when number three came along as well as my clinical work at that time, but I managed to get back to work when he was six months old. Sadly he had meningococcal septicaemia when he was ten weeks old so that put a spanner in the works, but we managed to live through that one and he is a very healthy boy. I sadly would say that work has strongly been at the forefront and I do feel that the family have coped and supported me because two part-time jobs do not equal one full-time job, I'd say they equal 1.5 jobs. There's some regret on my side in that I haven't been able to spend as much time with the children as I would have liked.

"Practicalities of childcare were that we used nurseries all the way through for the children with occasional use of childcare arrangements after school and before school. In latter years it hasn't been so much of an issue as the children are obviously bigger and the youngest is now nine years old and my husband has been extremely helpful taking him to school and picking him up from school. At one point when I was doing my research my childcare cost more than my salary, but that's something that other doctors who've worked part-time have experienced. So it was certainly not a financial gain to be working. My youngest son may consider going into medicine but the older two clearly do not approve of the hours of work and they just feel very strongly that that is not their career pathway. My oldest son is destined for a musical career and the second son is destined for some career associated with sport, so I don't really feel it's an issue."

Carol's outside interests include oboe-playing and keeping fit by means of aerobics, swimming and windsurfing.

"Unfortunately, I don't play in an orchestra at the present time, I would love to but time does not permit me to do that. I play the oboe annually at the Royal College of Paediatrics and Child Health Conference in York. The College has an orchestra which is pooled together from College members and we perform on an annual basis. I would like to join a local orchestra but at present I don't have any time. In terms of our family, my eldest son plays classical guitar and he also has a rock band. He is about to have his first performance on Oldham Street in Manchester, which I am allowed to attend, and my second son plays the flute. My second son and I are both learning the tin whistle at the present time, so we're learning some Irish music, which is really fun, and my youngest son has a drum kit and is planning to play percussion.

"My husband is a teacher, he is currently teaching English and Creative Writing in adult education on a part-time basis and he's managing domestic arrangements at home. His late father was a writer, you may remember someone called Edward Blishen who used to chair a programme called 'A Good Read' on a Sunday night on Channel 4, sadly he died three years ago. John has taken up the writing pen after the death of his father and he hopes to publish a book on working as a teacher in inner city Manchester, in the near future.

"In terms of my greatest professional challenge, I really feel my whole life has been a professional challenge and I can't really divide it up, I just meet each one as it comes along. I do feel that there are times, particularly in a situation where I've been a trainee, that senior doctors perceive me as being junior, and part-time has a certain feel to it which unfortunately is not eradicated as yet. I think probably my greatest disappointment was the attitude to me when I went for the interview for the PM79(3) scheme, in that clearly the interview panel were considering my application in a different light to my career aspirations and I did not feel as if that message was getting across. I didn't really know in retrospect how I would have done it differently. I think on the whole that the attitude to part-time work has improved to a degree but there still is an attitude that I come across as Associate Dean for Flexible Training, that it still gets referred to as the Married Woman's Part-Time Scheme and it's really not that. We have men, not a lot of men but some men on the scheme and we have very focused female trainees who are very clear in their career pathways, so I think we're getting away from it, but I think the culture of medicine does still allow that attitude to exist and we have to be very professional at how we eradicate it.

"Looking at the specialties, there are female doctors wanting to train across the board and I think it's very encouraging that at the present time we have flexible trainees training in surgery and other specialties where historically perhaps women haven't gone in to those specialties. I do feel that the culture is changing and that the specialties are seeing very committed trainees which does help their case enormously, so I do feel that the climate over the next five years will see some change.

"I don't regret going into medicine. I do have regrets about the amount of time it has taken up of my life, I do feel the balance between work and home and outside interests should be easier for people like myself. In reality, it's just not feasible, there just aren't enough hours in the day to get everything done, and unfortunately work always seems to come to the top as a priority.

Job-sharing. What can I say, it's my other 'marriage', I've been officially 'married' to Dr Eileen Baildam since 1988 and we're extremely good friends. We didn't know each other before we teamed up, again, our mentor Dr Barbara Phillips was the instigator in getting us together. It works exceedingly well, not only from a work point of view but as a way of giving support to each other and as consultants I feel this is something that is strongly lacking for consultants, that there aren't many opportunities for consultants to have support from colleagues in a way which is valued and which can be positive. So all in all it is good. I think the difficulty is that two half-time job-sharers equals probably 1.5 full-time equivalent doctors because you bring to the job your interests and your expertise, and when you combine them together that usually means more than one whole-time equivalent post. This does create difficulties and has created difficulties considerably for both of us at the present time, but all in all I would encourage it as a very good way of working and I would certainly look at possible job-shares, for example between doctors who wish to work part-time before they retire and junior doctors coming in at the other end. I see that as another way where organisations could have a flexible and effective workforce. At the moment I'm not doing too much about job-share initiatives but I hope as Associate Dean over the next year or two that I can help with any flexible workplace initiatives to encourage job-sharing. Furthermore, flexible working is an integral part of our workforce planning to recruit and retain staff. I would encourage both male and female senior doctors to consider jobsharing as they approach retirement."

Carol believes women can make a much greater contribution to medicine than is recognised at present. She advises girls considering medicine as a career not to be put off by stereotypic role models, to be fit and energetic and always willing to learn.

DR. MAIREAD ELLIS
General Practitioner

"I qualified at Sheffield University in 1983 and this was my first choice medical school. As far as the choice of medical school is concerned I wouldn't have made a different one. I actually made a decision to study medicine at the age of seven or eight and I think a lot of children at that age make a decision about careers that they don't necessarily stick to or keep. In my particular case it was a decision that my family wholeheartedly supported and that I was never really allowed to seriously question, so it was always assumed from that age that was what I was going to do. As far as being encouraged, as I've said at home I was very much encouraged to apply for medicine. At school, I went to a state school at the time but there was still in place a grammar school system, so I was in a convent grammar school and the ethos there was very much that we were good catholic girls being trained to be good catholic girls and therefore the only viable options in terms of career were motherhood, teaching or nursing. So they were somewhat discouraging about medicine.

"After qualifying, I had no difficulty in obtaining posts at house officer or SHO level in the required specialities for general practice which, however, had not been my original career choice, but it was one I felt was a practical one. In reality, if I'd been given a free choice in what I was going to do, I would actually have been a surgeon and probably second to that a psychiatrist. I received very little careers advice, but what I did was very discouraging about any sort of hospital career. Other than general practice the only other career that I was actively encouraged to consider was one in what was then community health, but now is really public health medicine rather than just straightforward baby clinic stuff. The career advice I was actually given all revolved around the fact that the choice of either community medicine or general practice was perceived as being very suitable for women who were either married or going to be married and certainly if they were anticipating having children."

Mairead got married six months before qualifying but did not start her family until seven years later. She has had to rely on paid childcare and still finds it difficult to reconcile the demands of work and the family. She says, "It has taken me a long time to separate, emotionally, work from outside life. I feel the things that make me a good doctor are the very things that drain and burn me out."

She has considered quitting medicine and saw a careers counsellor quite recently, but has decided to continue as a GP until her children are independent, then find work overseas with VSO or MSF.

"I have lots of interests outside medicine aside from bringing up three children, particularly music and the arts. I am currently two-thirds the way through an Open University BA which is in music and European humanities. The time for this really now is because I work part-time, because I decided that I needed something outside of medicine, some form of relaxation, some time for me and studying with the Open University fitted in with my lifestyle in that it's difficult to go out at night with the children. So, if I'm going to be in the house, it's easier to be doing or I find it more enjoyable to be doing that than just sat in front of the telly all night. Working part-time, yes, does have a financial implication. I'm actually divorced so from a financial point of view I live in a smaller house than I used to when I was married, but I live in a house that I can afford and am happy with. Working part-time, it's really not the money that's the most important thing, it's having the time to spend time doing things for the children, feeling I'm fulfilling my maternal role as well and that I have time for me as an individual, not just me as a GP who everybody else comes and makes demands on.

"When I had the children, I had thirteen weeks standard maternity leave. Within our partnership agreement thirteen weeks was the allocated time period because that was the time that the FHSA were reimbursing locum costs, albeit at a fairly pathetic rate. I probably could have persuaded my partner to let me take more time off work, but financially I couldn't have afforded that because that would have been unpaid. I also had some difficulty in my last period of maternity leave when my partners decided that they thought I'd had too many children too quickly and they decided four weeks before I went off to have my third child that, rather than spread the additional locum costs between the partners, they were going to charge it all to me which led to a great deal of unhappiness and aggro within the practice, even to the extent of me actually seeking legal advice about what was going on. Fortunately, they backed down but that was not a particularly pleasant thing to be going through at the same time as being thirty-six weeks pregnant, diabetic and feeling thoroughly fed up with life.

"Yes, coping with home and children is difficult to fit in with work. It's easier working part-time, but there are difficulties in finding reliable childcare where the children are happy and it's particularly difficult in school holidays, because certainly at the moment when my children are at school they go to before-and-after-school club and they're reasonably tolerant of that. When it's school holidays and there's whole days when they have to be there they get very resentful. Fortunately during the summer holidays my mother has them for a week and takes them off to Norfolk so in that sense I rely on that and so do they for at least a break over the summer holidays.

"It's difficult to say what is the greatest professional challenge I've had to meet. There's always a certain degree of satisfaction and challenge in dealing with individual particular patients and getting it right for them, but overall in my professional career I think the biggest challenge is that things are constantly changing. Patients obviously present different problems every time they come in, which is change, but also the structure of general practice as it exists has changed really ever since I became a principal in 1988 which was just before the 1990 contract. Since then, everything's been on the move. As far as professional achievements are concerned it would be easy to say passing various exams, except I don't really see them as great achievements, just hoops to be jumped through. From my point of view I think at the moment the thing that pleases me most is that over the last four or five years in my practice we've managed to get together a like-minded team and built what we hope is a fairly effective, happy primary healthcare team and I see that as being one of the biggest achievements that I've actually played a part in. As far as disappointment is concerned I think the biggest disappointment for me is finding how many people are now very cynical about the whole process and therefore very unwilling to engage in anything, just seeing everything as a waste of time and doomed to failure.

"As to how I rate the NHS: I believe certainly for the money invested in it the NHS is an excellent service. I think on the whole it's got dedicated hard-working staff who rise to most of the challenges presented to them. However, it's difficult sometimes, certainly for me and I think for a lot of people working in the NHS to understand how the system and the services are perceived by users. We assume what's happening and what we believe to be happening to be the case where it would appear that a lot of people are dissatisfied because we're not actually doing what we think we are. For example, we think we run an efficient appointments system within our practice so we actually do meet targets like, if patients need to be seen urgently they can and will be seen that day. Patients' perception of our service seems to be more that, when they demand it, it should happen and they have no comprehension or understanding of the fact that if they are demanding an emergency appointment and if there's ten of them, that's an extra hour on someone's surgery, an extra hour of their time which is either taken out of other work or out of their own personal lives.

"In terms of the greatest challenges for medicine: I would see two big areas of challenge; one is in academic medicine, in perhaps developing new drugs for cancer or in the highly academic research arena. Perhaps I would say the greatest challenges for public health, which includes some aspects of medicine, are more social changes, behaviour pattern changes, so that the effects that smoking for instance, poverty, social deprivation have on the health of the nation are all reduced.

"Anything men doctors can do, women doctors can do, probably even better. A lot of the skills required as a practising doctor are skills that are traditionally associated and ascribed to women. It doesn't necessarily mean that women are any better at them, but they start out with a better chance anyway. Having said that, the intellectual and academic side of medicine is something that women are equally capable of and they should be encouraged, if they want, to go down that line rather than just to be seen as hands-on workers.

"I found and joined the MWF at a time when I was getting very little support professionally from partners and other people around me. So that belonging to the MWF, just knowing that there's an organisation there that is much more supportive, that does allow for meeting other women who are struggling with some of the same problems, has been very, very useful.

"For young people contemplating medicine as a career, I think there is still a sort of aura around medicine as a career as being a wonderful thing to do for very altruistic motives. Whilst I'm not denying that is a part of medicine, I think that anybody who is going to be doing that for the next forty years of their lives needs to seriously look at what it is they enjoy and what it is they want to get out of their working life and if they enjoy working hard, working with people, meeting constant change and all the challenges involved in that, then medicine could well be a very satisfying career, but it's not easy."

MRS AKMAL SIDDIQUI
Ophthalmologist

Akmal qualified in Manchester in 1984. She grew up in Leigh in Lancashire; her mother was a GP and her father was a barrister. The choice of medicine as a career was only partly her own as she was strongly encouraged to become a doctor both at home and at her state school, Leigh Girls' Grammar School. When she did not get into Cambridge, which had been her first choice, she opted for Manchester and has never wished she had been anywhere else.

Akmal married a fellow doctor three years after qualifying and had her first child within a year, which was unplanned, but not regretted. A second followed two years later, then a third after a gap of nine years. She took between four and nine months off work after her confinements. She has used both paid childcare and family help, and says her parents have been the greatest support of all.

A career in ophthalmology was always her ambition but the training was so difficult to fit in with bringing up her children that for a time she considered switching to general practice. She took a career break of over three years and it was the greatest challenge she has faced to start operating again, but in the end she has surmounted all the obstacles and become a consultant ophthalmologist in Wigan. Obtaining her Fellowship and consultant post have been the professional achievements which have pleased her most.

Akmal switched to part-time training after starting her family, but points out the disadvantages of this route. It will inevitably take twice as long to complete one's training and if one is supernumerary, as Akmal was in an early post in Manchester, there can be a problem about accumulating sufficient experience. This is particularly the case in a surgical specialty where there is competition for "cutting." However, there are flexible training posts where the part-timer is nevertheless treated as a true member of the team and Akmal found a post like this in Liverpool which was much more satisfactory. The quality of supervision along the way has also been disappointing at times, and colleague support not always as good as it should be.

On top of these vicissitudes, Akmal feels that doctors are poorly paid for all their hard work, and that women doctors are undervalued. Although she has now reached her goal of becoming a consultant there are new strains to face with huge responsibilities and pressure to lengthen operating lists. She advises young people considering a career in medicine to think carefully and find out as much as possible by meeting a lot of young doctors in different specialties.

DR. REBECCA BARON
General Practitioner

"I trained in Manchester and qualified in 1984. During medical school I wasn't terribly involved or terribly organised in anything, and just sort of went through. It was my first choice of medical school, I think partly because I wanted to come to Manchester, not because I particularly liked it, in fact when I came to look round I thought it was not particularly attractive but came nevertheless. I think it was a very big year and that was probably a bit of a down side to it, and quite a lot of didactic teaching which I'm pleased to see is now changing. So in terms of whether I wish I'd gone to a different one, occasionally I think I might have preferred to have gone to one with a more integrated syllabus and at the time when I was looking I think Leicester had, and Newcastle had, but I didn't particularly want to go to those places, so overall I've no regrets, because I'm happy where I am now.

"It was my decision to study medicine, my dad was quite keen for me to do it and I was quite keen on doing biochemistry, due to influence of a boyfriend at the time, which then changed to medicine so it was all a bit hit-and-miss, really. I think I went into medicine thinking I wanted to be a geneticist which is quite bizarre when I look back on it now, I was going to do medicine and then do something else. So it was my decision and I did really, I think, ultimately want to work with people. In terms of whether there are other doctors in the family, there is, my grandfather was a doctor but I didn't get on with him and in fact I think he would have put me off rather than encouraged me. He had been a GP and he hated general practice, he thought it was the lowest of the low. He was a psychiatrist and thought that was the only thing that was worth doing. He was one of the few people I never really got on particularly well with, so yes, there was a doctor in the family, but I don't think that was a factor.

"Did I have any discouragement? From home definitely no, my family were very keen. My dad who was supposed to become a dentist but in fact went into business and then became a writer, couldn't bear the sight of blood and hated doctors but wanted me to be one and school were very supportive. I was in a direct grant, so had a free place at an independent school, which was very fortunate for me. After qualifying I organised house jobs and then got on a rotation at Stepping Hill. I was quite fortunate in my surgical house job, the registrar I worked with had been a GP and gone back into surgery and he was really supportive and helpful in terms of applying and interviewing. I was quite pleased to get that post because at that time there was quite a lot of competition and I was quite keen to come back to Stockport.

"In terms of field of medicine, having done a GP training post I went straight into general practice. I actually really liked obstetrics and did think I might go back and do obstetrics after my trainee year but I quickly changed my mind having got into general practice. The other field of medicine I have worked in really from the first year of going into general practice was being involved in education. I was a Course Organiser in Stockport for the day release course and was really very fortunate to do that and to work with somebody who taught me a lot about education, and in my trainee year, worked again with someone who was always very involved in education and really got me sort of fired up in terms of what could be done and making changes. That was really exciting because it was quite an innovative scheme and we made quite a lot of developments in terms of integrating General Practice Training into the hospital part of the jobs and that was really good. I did that for quite a number of years, in fact I think about eight years altogether.

"Then about seven years ago, a group of us had been on a training course, a Leadership Course that the MSD Foundation used to run and we really enjoyed it, I did it probably about a year or two after I'd been in practice, and it was really a group based course, group work and it was quite important for me in giving me confidence. I can remember going on that course being a bit embarrassed saying I was a Course Organiser because I knew I was so young to be doing it and I thought they were all going to laugh at me, and really at the end of the course which went on over about eighteen months I felt a lot more confident in terms of what I was doing and that was really, really helpful. One of the other things that you covered was a lot about developing your practice and how to institute change. We'd all felt similarly about it and there were no courses like that running subsequently. What happened was a few of us got together and thought we ought to have courses like that in the Region again and with support from Region we ran a couple of courses. They were each three day courses, three modules per course, looking at personal development, practice development and professional development and they were great, a really rewarding part of what I've done. They went very well, the feedback was great and we really enjoyed doing them, it was just really nice to work with people and feel motivated. The sort of feedback from the course was that people felt very motivated, because I think people feel so bogged down with what they're doing, there's no time, they know changes need to happen, but it's kind of where do you begin and it just gave people time to stand back and look and think about it. As a result of that and also a change in the National Agenda there's been more support and we had a lot more support from Region to set up. I've been involved in higher professional training for GPs which is based on those courses but also has a day a month study day, quite a lot of management training, and is accredited towards MSc level. It's in modules so people can do a year or a year and a half and if they want they can get a certificate in general practice, whatever that means, they can go on and do further modules and get a diploma, and they can go on and get an MSc. It's not about encouraging people to do unnecessary qualifications but it's actually about acknowledging the level of work that people are doing. I spend three sessions a week officially doing higher professional training so that fits quite well really because it's quite flexible. I run three residentials a year with three days each that I'm away for, and then I have eight teaching days a year and we have quite a lot of meetings in-between of the tutors, but a lot of the work I do in my own time is quite flexible. I do a lot of work at weekends when it suits me which I like. We've written a course book for the course, I've written longish chapters on quite a range of management topics and other areas so it's been quite interesting in that respect, and it makes me realise I need to do some more work on my writing skills but that's good fun, so that's part of what I do. So that's the sort of educational field I work in. I stopped course organising a few years ago because doing both was getting a bit much.

"Then I have a third aspect to what I do and as a result of taking on the third aspect, I've gone three-quarter time in general practice and that is working on PCG Groups. I'm Clinical Governance lead for our PCG Group and I'm very involved at the moment in the proposal for a Trust for Stockport, the Primary Care Trust, and that's been really interesting, a completely different aspect to what I've done before, working in a kind of management large organisation and seeing how large organisations work and how different they are to General Practice. I suppose for that it's probably worked out about a couple, it's supposed to be about a session and a half a week or maybe two sessions a week but in fact practice ends up vast amounts more than that. It's quite interesting because it's not as intensive as General Practice in any way, but it takes quite a long time to do the stuff and one of the things I've learnt in my education side is that if you want to make a change you have to sit down and do it and write it, it's no good just going to a meeting and talking about it, and you then actually have to get things implemented. My Clinical Governance side, the area that I've led on, is getting together a protected time scheme for Stockport which seems to be going well, so that practices can have half a day out four times a year as a practice to discuss issues, and half a day four times a year when they meet with other practices to have workshops and introductions to areas. Practice-wise I'm, say, three-quarter time. The practice I joined was just myself and another doctor, but we've actually taken on, a couple of years ago, a third doctor which has enabled me to go three-quarter time and it's a very supportive practice. My partners are very supportive of the other work I do.

"Did I have a career plan? I think I did want to go into general practice fairly soon, I think I thought that was probably what would suit me. I had one good experience in Medical School with an attachment near Rochdale and one rather miserable appointment somewhere else at home which really wasn't very encouraging but I did know that wasn't the norm. The education, I think, once I got involved in it, I realised that it was something that I really wanted to do and although I have kind of seized the opportunity I think it's been my long term aim to get further involved in that. So I have changed my mind a bit I suppose because I did think I might go back to obstetrics but mainly I've kept along the same route.

"Principal interests outside? I've got lots really. I do lots of theatre visiting, opera, music and I'm really keen on gardening – I've got a large garden – and walking, outdoor skiing, I like being outside a lot of the time, friends, entertaining, lots of things really, there's not enough hours in the day. I'm not married, I've lived with somebody for about six years, I have a partner. He's not a doctor, he's actually now retired but he was a computer programmer, it's wonderful to have your own in-house IT Department, I strongly recommend it. I don't have any children.

"The greatest professional challenge I've had to meet? I think for me personally it's actually clinical uncertainty – that's the thing I've found the hardest and I still find the hardest. I go through kind of waxes and wanes really, it's that that keeps me awake at night. I don't lie awake at night worrying about meetings and what people have said to me etcetera in terms of education and management, it's really the patients, if I'm worried I should have done something or might have missed something or whatever, and that's my own personal thing. I find that as long as I'm not working too flat out I cope with it quite well but if I'm doing too much clinical work and I'm really working flat out and I don't have time to stop and think, I get home at night and think, I'm not very happy. So that's been my own personal thing.

"Professional achievements that have pleased me most? I think getting the Higher Professional Training course up and running and the feedback from that, it's just so lovely. I mean every year we take about 24 people and you just get to know them really well in the group, and it is so nice to just talk to people about actually what you do, because you go to meetings and you have these kind of superficial moaning conversations about this, that and the other, but actually to talk about work and what it really means in the relationship with patients, and just see people sort problems out, not necessarily sort them but actually, we've had people come who've been in really difficult practices, and I wouldn't say they'd solved it but it's stopped bugging them as much – that's been really, really nice. I got an FRCGP and I got a big boost out of that actually, I must admit, it was really nice, that.

"What is the greatest disappointment in my career? I can't think of one. No, I haven't got any.

"How do I rate the NHS? Fair to good really. I think it could be a lot better, I'd like to think that the National Plan is not as my partner suggested a work of fiction. There was some complaining about reading it in bed, I don't normally read work in bed, and he said, 'It's okay because it's only fiction anyway,' but I think it is good and I think there's such a lot of really good people who work in it who are very dedicated, and I think motivation and time out for personal development would have a big impact on improvement of things. I think more funding's required but overall I think it's a pretty sound basis, and if the funding's there to do what needs to be done, things could get an awful lot better.

"What do I regard as the greatest challenge? I think good organisation and good management, the right management, so I think good management but not wasting money on management that isn't right, and I think the vital part in that is clinical leadership in management, because I think if you're not actually working in the area you don't have very close contact. It's too easy to write documents and plan things and not actually implement them, and I think that's what's happened a lot of the time. I think coping with all that's new, the changes in healthcare and what needs to be done, and the sort of changes in ways we can treat people and acknowledging that that is actually a lot more work, and really providing good one-to-one basic communication to patients and good care, those are the challenges.

"The contribution of women doctors I think is high, I would say that because I think they are very good communicators, men have got a lot to offer as well but certainly women doctors have got a lot and I think the options for working flexibly are there. Although I suppose I'm three-quarter time in practice, if I work out the number of hours I do it's like other people's full-time but then I suppose if you look at managers who are doing jobs on similar salaries, they do hours that are long, that's part of the way it goes, but I think there is a lot of flexibility and opportunity to be involved in other things, certainly I enjoy having different aspects to my job, that really keeps me interested.

"How have I been influenced by belonging to the MWF? I've read the information that comes out and just realise, I suppose, I've been very lucky because I don't think I've ever felt in any way discriminated against, I think probably because I don't have children. I think maybe that makes things more difficult when you're more limited in time and I think it's important that things like that are discussed.

"What advice would I offer? I think I would say it can be a really rewarding job, I think there's lots of options for things you can do and I think to me to do a job that you actually feel can make a difference is very important to me. It is hard work but I think a lot of things you want to do are and that's where you get your rewards from."

DR. SUSAN FOX
Neurology Specialist Registrar

Susan's decision to study medicine was encouraged both at home and at her school, which was in the state system. She qualified at Manchester University Medical School in 1990.

"My first choice for medical school was actually to go to Cambridge because that's where my dad went, and I felt I was sort of as a family obliged to apply there because my grandfather also went and my great-uncle, so it was a bit of a family tradition. However, needless to say, I didn't get in and in the end I was quite pleased I went to Manchester.

"Yes, there were other doctors in my family. There was my great-aunt Alice who lived in Cambridge and was a Cambridge institution, she was rather eccentric, even in her late eighties, early nineties, lived in blue overalls and wellington boots and used to take in waifs, not literally waifs and strays but overseas students who had nowhere to stay in Cambridge. She lived fairly near the University campus. She was a doctor at Newnham College, which was an all-female college, at the beginning of the century and was one of the first female doctors there and she ended up doing child psychiatry. She was quite a prominent figure when I was a youngster, we used to go and stay with her and she used to terrify me because she used to make me eat artichokes which I absolutely hated and the house was always in such a state, it was never clean, there was dust completely everywhere and I always thought, well, if she can be a doctor and do all this then it must be a good career.

"I ended up doing neurology really because it was the one aspect of medicine that really fascinated me. I remember watching a video as a second year medical student, one of the neurologists had brought a video in of all these people with funny movements and I was really taken with these people with their arms flinging everywhere, because it's such a visual specialty, that was really one of the things that I liked. The other thing is it's fairly challenging anatomically when you have a patient with a neurological condition, trying to figure out where the lesion is, and I quite liked that, it's sort of almost like a detective story as you work your way down and think, 'Ah yes, well it can't be this, it's got to be that,' and when it all clicks together it's quite satisfying. So I think that's why I ended up in neurology. I clearly went down the medicine line because I absolutely hated surgery. I detested standing in theatre with the retractors for hours and hours and hours and I had a horrible experience as a fourth-year medical student when the consultant I worked with disappeared out of theatre and said, "You can sew up," and I was left with this abdomen to stitch up. Luckily I'd done a little bit of stitching but I was absolutely petrified trying to stitch this abdomen up and I decided that was it, surgery was not for me."

Susan believes women have a lot to offer as doctors, being generally better organised and more caring than the men. She has not experienced any gender discrimination thus far. "After qualifying I've not had any problems obtaining posts because I'm a woman, clearly I haven't got every single job I've gone to but that's sort of the competition and I don't think I've really ever come across any brick walls or glass ceilings at the moment anyway. I've got the final hurdle to come so things might change!

"How were the work hours and work rotas that I did? My first house job was fairly onerous, I worked on the renal transplant unit at Manchester Royal Infirmary and there were three house officers and we basically did a one-in-three which went down to a one-in-two when somebody was off on holiday, but that was clearly the worst rota I did. I remember working two weeks and having one night off in that two weeks. I mean it doesn't sound as bad as people used to do many years ago but the amount of work that we had to do then is probably more than perhaps people used to do thirty, forty years ago. So that was fairly hectic. After that my average rota would be a one-in-five or one-in-six on-call and generally sort of nine-to-five in most jobs. The worst job I did was another renal job at Manchester Royal Infirmary where I rarely left the ward before six or even seven at night on a regular basis, so that was fairly wearing, but I think in neurology hours-wise it's fairly civilised, it's again reasonably nine-to-five. The on-call rota I do currently is a one-in-six non-residential and you're very unlucky if you get called in at night or at the weekends, so it's very manageable. So I think overall I haven't really had any major problem with my rota or the hours particularly, not for any prolonged period, just sort of short periods. The argument the surgeons always give is that if you don't put the hours in then you really don't get the training, so there's got to be a balance and overall I'm fairly happy with what I did.

"Regarding the greatest challenges for medicine in the future. One that's fairly close to my heart having done a PhD looking at potential new treatments for things like Parkinson's disease, we can make great leaps forward in scientific discoveries and hopefully identify new treatments but then it's actually taking it up into clinical use that I think is going to be one of the biggest challenges because there's only a finite budget that the NHS has and clearly new drugs are going to be limited, they're not all going to be fully beneficial for everybody so I think this is going to be one of the big challenges. As we've ascertained the full human genome now there's going to be more and more discoveries made, patients' groups will clearly be advocating for new drugs and I think if this is all going to cause major problems, I suppose the argument could be that we just stop the scientific discoveries now, because what's the point if you can't get the drugs into the market place. Again, I think gene therapy is something that's going to come more and more into actual daily clinical practice, I think these things are definitely going to be around in the next 10-20 years and the challenges are going to be the cost of them on the background of all the sort of general day-to-day costs that the NHS has to cover.

"What advice would I offer to a young person contemplating medicine as a career? My feeling about this is that you're never really told what it's like on a day-to-day basis being a doctor, you might perhaps see it on the television in soap operas but it's obviously different to what it's like in real life. They don't show you how tired you get, how difficult it can be dealing with ten things all at once, bleeps going off, not getting your food at regular mealtimes, going home feeling tired, not wanting to do anything and obviously social life suffering. So I think it's important that people actually visit a hospital or a GP surgery and actually spend not just a day, probably a few days with a doctor over several hours per day just really seeing what the continual pressures are, seeing the negative side but also obviously to see the positive side and just to see what a challenging job it can be. Because I went into medicine not really understanding, I don't think, what it was like to be a doctor, I don't think at the age of eighteen you have really an idea of what it's like. I mean you know what a builder does and you know what a milkman does but a doctor, it's different, because it's not something that people come across in day-to-day lives. You may obviously see your GP as a child if you go in ill with something but you clearly don't see the other side of what the job is actually like."

Susan says she has not yet had time to start a family. Her partner is not a doctor. Their favourite interests are travelling to exotic locations and eating out. The professional achievement which has pleased her most was obtaining her PhD. In the year 2001 Susan has completed her higher professional training and has obtained a consultant appointment at the Walton Centre for Neurology and Neurosurgery, Liverpool, thus clearing her final hurdle with flying colours.

DR. NGOZI EDI-OSAGIE
Neonatal Paediatrics Specialist Registrar

Ngozi started life in Manchester but when she was ten her father's job with Mobil Oil took the family to Nigeria, where she completed her education.

"I went to Benin Medical School in Nigeria and I qualified in 1990. Why did I do medicine? I did it because my mum is a nurse and my dad was an engineer, but in Nigeria you've got to do a profession and if you're good at science in school then you're told to do medicine and if you're good at arts you do law. If you're female they tend to say do medicine because engineering is left for the men. So I ended up doing medicine because I was good at the sciences in secondary school when I was doing my O-levels. Benin was the first medical school of my choice, my dad wanted me to go to a different one because there was one that was very good and this was okay, but this had a better social life, the one I went to, so it would be like sort of the Manchester University of Nigeria, that's what it would be like, because it had a really good social life and so I did want to go. They had a university that is one of the oldest universities with the oldest medical school and that is where he wanted me to go, but I didn't end up going there. I didn't wish I went to a different one because I met my husband at university and I have lots of friends that I still keep in touch with, and it was right in the middle of Nigeria so was easily accessible to lots of places so I liked that.

"Doing medicine was partly my own decision because you don't have, well, you do have people that inherit money in Nigeria but not a lot, and you're really driven by the will to succeed and so everybody wants to do a profession. If you don't go to university it is because your family couldn't afford it, there's nobody that would have the chance to go and not go so it was my own decision, I knew I wanted to do a profession and medicine seemed like a good idea. I had no discouragement whatsoever from either home or school but lots of encouragement. There are no other doctors in the family but Mum's a nurse, so we did have lots of friends that had parents that were doctors because of the fact that she was a nurse. I was born in Manchester and I grew up in Manchester and she used to work at Crumpsall Hospital, my mum, and was friendly with lots of the foreign doctors. We had lots of friends come over to the house and like I wear my wristwatch on my right hand because a doctor once told me, I think I was about seven, that doctors wear their wristwatches on their right hand to take the pulse so I've always worn it on my right hand from when I was about seven. I found out that's not true, but…

"I went to a private boarding school from the age of ten and after qualifying my dad died when I was a house officer and my mum's West Indian so she came back to England. So I did most of my house jobs and then I came to England and I did PLAB, because my mum was here with my brothers and sisters because her mother, my grandmother, lives in Manchester so she came back to be near her family. It so happened I was in the library one day and I met the consultant that I did my electives with and he said, "Well, why not come and do an attachment?" So while I was reading for PLAB I used to go to the unit twice a week and join in the ward rounds. Then after I passed PLAB he gave me a reference and the first job I applied for, I got it. I haven't had any problems obtaining posts throughout my career, it's always been okay, I haven't had any difficulties, I think mainly because I usually applied for things that were appropriate. Because on the day it's also dependent on how many people they want, so I've been lucky that there's been no PhD thesis person that wants six months of paediatrics when I was applying, so my career's been fairly straightforward.

"I've always done paediatrics and in Nigeria you don't have paediatric patients that have long-term chronic illnesses. So one of the main reasons why I did paediatrics when I was going through medical school is because paediatric case notes were really short. I remember coming to England and the first paediatric job I got was on Acorn ward and you have really big case notes. In Nigeria if you have chronic illnesses you don't survive. So in adult medicine you'd have people who would have things come in and go out but paediatric patients, you were either well or you were not well and died. That was the main reason why I chose paediatrics and plus I did like the doctors that were in paediatrics. I never changed my mind, I've always wanted to do paediatrics. When I started paediatrics I did two years of general and specialty paediatrics and then I did neonates for six months, and as soon as I did neonates I knew I wanted to do neonates. So I've never deviated from what I wanted to do because before that I didn't have any strong feelings about what specialty I was going to do, some specialty within paediatrics, because if I'd done general paediatrics I would have liked to have a special interest in something. So I did neonates and I liked that and that's what I've done since then.

"My principal outside interest is travel. I try and visit a new country every year so I can see as many as I can before I go, so that's my principal interest.

"I got married three years after I qualified. My husband is a doctor, he's a year five SpR in obstetrics and his career has been fairly straightforward as well, we've always managed to get jobs, because in Manchester, being in the North West, there are lots of hospitals. So as SHO's we didn't have problems, we worked together, and as registrars you get a rotation so we've been lucky in that way. My daughter was born five years after I qualified and that was planned, we planned that we wouldn't have any children until we passed our exams so I passed mine, I did my exams in February and his exams were in May. My membership was in February and his membership was in May. After I passed mine I said, 'Well we might as well start trying,' and he said, 'We already agreed…' but I thought, 'Well, it never happens straightaway so we'll just try,' and it happened straightaway. So I was about two months pregnant when he passed his exams, but thank God he passed because it's hard work doing it with children. After she came I realised how much hard work it would have been if we hadn't had our exams before she came.

"I took six months off and I wouldn't have changed the timing because I think it's very difficult to do as an SHO. If SHO's have children there are not many SHO's that are part-time, you tend to get your SHO jobs out of the way and become part-time as a registrar. So it's almost impossible to live a good family life and do a shift system as most of the jobs are now at SHO level, so I think I wouldn't have changed it at all, when she was born, when we decided to do it.

"As for coping with home and children, it hasn't been too difficult for me. I have a very supportive partner, and my mum lives here, I've got aunties and uncles, I've got all my brothers and sisters in Manchester. When she was first born, after I went back to work my mother-in-law came and stayed for six months so she didn't actually go to nursery until she was a year and I felt it still was very hard, I used to sit in the car-park every day and cry after I'd dropped her off. It was still hard, but at least I felt she was a bit older so she could cope with being out of the house. I thought it was too difficult to wake them up when they were very young and take them out into the cold and take them to the nursery, but if you've got to do it, then you've got to do it. She was a bit older when we had to start doing that and we were both registrars, we were both in jobs that we were doing one in five on-call and one in six so we could always make sure we weren't on-call on the same day and so that helped. For days we want off, Mum will come and take her for a day at the weekend or an evening when we're really too tired, so I've coped because I've had lots of family around. We've paid for childcare all along but it's one of the things you've got to do. She went to a nursery, we didn't have a nanny, I didn't feel comfortable with the idea of having one sole person with my child during the day. I liked the idea of the nursery and it was very near to where I was working, very near to Hope, it was about two minutes away so I could go across or phone up, so that was nice.

"Is my child going to follow me into medicine? She is only five, but hopefully not, to tell the truth. I really wouldn't want her to, because I enjoy what I do but I think it takes a big chunk of your life. My sister is a solicitor, she is five years younger than me and never works weekends, she earns more than me, she's got her own secretary. Before you get to the end which I suppose would be consultant you're in your mid-thirties and a lot of time has gone and then, even after that, especially now with all the paperwork, it's not ended, so I don't want her to have this sort of life. I can do it because I enjoy what I do, but I think I'd like her to do something so that she had enough money to enjoy herself and have a nice life. I want her to have a nice life, I wouldn't describe my life as nice. It must get better, I'm sure, when you settle down in one place, I think it's the uncertainty of where you're going to end up, where you're going to get consultant jobs — we have to get them in the same town, in the same region. When we were at university people would say, 'Well, at least you're sure of a job when you're a doctor.' But then I have friends that didn't do medicine, and they did other things, some are journalists and they go all over the world and they seem to have such an interesting life. I don't know, I don't know what I want for her, unless she's really determined to do it, unless she's really, really keen, I don't want her to do it. I don't want her to do it because she thinks 'I'll always have a job,' or 'It's nice being a doctor.' I don't want her to do it if that's the case, she's got to be really keen. I think it helps if you're clever because there was one great disappointment in my career and that was when I did my MRCP and I didn't pass and that was the first exam I hadn't passed. I just felt sick, I don't know, lots of people have setbacks, but I don't know what it was, I didn't like the idea that I had to do it again, your life's stopped, everything revolves around this exam. I didn't feel ashamed, I just felt that so much effort and energy and time had gone into this, I remember I was in London at the time and I couldn't go out, well you could but every time you went out you felt guilty about the time you were supposed to be devoting to reading for this exam, so the exams – I didn't like them.

"My professional achievements: an award I got from the Royal Society of Medicine in 1997 was the achievement that has pleased me the most. My greatest professional challenge: what I find most challenging is trying to work with people that I think are intolerant. I find that a very great challenge, to not either rise to the occasion or do something about it. In my time, when I worked as an SHO with a registrar or nurses that were very intolerant and bigoted, I found that a very great challenge. Usually I try and get on, because there's not much you can do to change people, and sometimes you think because you're only there for six months you're not going to make any great changes. The other day we had an away day on the ward, on the neonatal unit, and I overheard one of the sisters asking, 'Are any of the SHO's coming, and she said, 'They're not part of the unit, they only stay here for six months, they're not members of staff,' and I think that's how they're viewed because we're all passing through and so it's not really your unit. But at Hope some of the nurses only stay for six months because there is a very high turnover in specialties that are high-intensity. Sometimes you think, "Why bother?" because you are only going to be here for six months so even though you meet this attitude that you're just passing through, you don't make any great changes especially as an SHO. As a registrar I did, if I went somewhere I thought it was my unit and I felt I had things to give, but that's what I've found most challenging. In day-to-day work you'll always meet either a difficult case or difficult parents or things but I consider that to be part of my job.

"How do I rate the NHS? Well, I've given it a pass mark, I gave it six out of ten because there's room for improvement, there's lots of room for improvement. The greatest challenges for the future are, I think, trying to get the balance between delivering healthcare and innovation and research especially in the light of what's been happening recently. I think we can get left behind and there must be funding available for research and proper guidelines and controls.

"How do I rate the contribution women doctors can make? I think we need to get involved in all areas of medicine. There are some areas in which it's very difficult to arrange a family around the work so that they're seen as male-dominated areas where there are not many women doctors. I think it would be nice if we got involved in all areas of medicine but above that, those specialties where there are not that many women should try and make it a bit more female-friendly and look at the problems as to why there are no females there. I haven't had such a problem because I've only got the one child and I've got family support, but it can be very difficult trying to juggle family and childcare, that must be the bane of most female doctors, I think that is the worst thing. The other reason why I didn't become a flexible trainee, I think it's changed a bit, when I first started when I was an SHO, the flexible trainees were always seen as an extra, they were never given any responsibility, they were never really part of the team and I didn't want to be like that, I really didn't. They just seemed to be an appendage because if a unit was supposed to run on three registrars they were delegated all the tasks and the flexible trainee wasn't given anything to do, because they were there as an addition and in the next six months there wouldn't be a flexible trainee, so they didn't really have a role. It's changed a bit now, I think it now depends on the person, I feel that depending on what you want to do you can go and demand that, 'I want to have this sort of training, I want this input, I want this to do,' so it has changed and again they're making most of the jobs into jobshares at registrar level now. It is good news, I think it's better because the other thing is there is a lot of resentment from full-timers to flexible trainees, because a flexible trainee can arrive and say, 'I'm only going to do Monday on-call.' Yes, it fits in with your childcare but some of the people that do full-time, male and female, have children too and you're being paid for one day a week and I'm being paid for two days a week, I can't choose my days, if I could I would. So now they've made them jobshares you're just another person but you split the on-call and then you arrange childcare around that so you can't say, 'I want this, this and this,' and just take all the nice bits and leave all the bad bits, so I think it is better that it's a jobshare.

"What advice would I offer to young people contemplating medicine as a career? I think you need to have dedication, you've got to be dedicated, you've got to be honest and you've got to be determined, because everybody has points where they'll face some sort of setback and it's not because you're not good, it just might be that you're unfortunate at that point in time. There might be jobs that I've applied for, if you had people there that were much better qualified then I wouldn't have got the job on that day, so there is some luck but you can help yourself along. A number of times I've done interviews at Hope and you have people that are totally unprepared or they send you a shoddy CV, if you really want the job why send in a shoddy CV that's not going to get you shortlisted? It makes me wonder sometimes why people don't make an effort at all if they really want something, it's either they don't really want it or they just can't be bothered."

DR. FIONA BLACKHALL
Oncology Specialist Registrar

I qualified in Manchester in 1992 after spending my preclinical years at St Andrews University where I also did an intercalated BSc. The contrast of these universities has been a great bonus. I went to a state school in Aberdeen and chose St Andrews/Manchester because I liked the idea of going 'South of the border.' We were advised to put Edinburgh first on our UCCA forms and I was offered a place but turned it down. They sent letters for several years asking why I had rejected them! I was quite shocked at St Andrews to find people assuming that I had been rejected from other universities. I became aware of the Oxbridge obsession and have been intrigued ever since. At school I thought these universities only did arts degrees! However I hate the assumption that graduates of these universities are better. I hope this changes during the next millennium because I think there is still an unhealthy bias towards those from the 'golden triangle' in hospital based specialities and academic medicine in particular.

Why did I decide to study medicine? I'm not really sure, I think it might have been those 'Your life in their hands' documentaries of the late 70's. I loved those documentaries and was allowed to stay up late to watch them. So when I was eight or nine I got the notion that I was going to do medicine (surgery in fact) and then found out what I needed to do. I was able to tell the teachers what I was aiming for and chose school subjects accordingly. Looking back I benefited greatly from having a goal at an early age. I'm naturally quite lazy at times academically and I don't think I would have done so well at school without a goal, particularly since the careers advice we received was abysmal. I remember many friends who could have gone to university but didn't because the teachers left it up to individuals to express an interest to go. I left school with straight A's but started university believing that I would struggle to keep up. I have subsequently become aware of a different philosophy in the independent schools and often feel angry that the teachers at our school were so discouraging. I had a bee in my bonnet about medicine and thankfully ignored them but I remember being told that medicine would be a very hard career for a woman. My family were supportive but I also remember my grandfather saying that I should do pharmacy so that I could run a shop and combine this with having children and I remember my mum saying, because I did lots of ballet and highland dancing classes, that I could always become a highland dancing teacher if I didn't get into medical school. I relied on the availability of a full grant to go to University and doubt whether I could have gone without that funding. I hope that children from lower income families are not put off medicine due to the changes in funding for students.

So how did I get into oncology? I did an SHO post in cardiac and respiratory medicine at Wythenshawe and part of that was working in the pulmonary oncology unit. Actually, before that, as a medical student, I was taught by a psychiatrist, Peter Maguire, who has spent his working life researching and teaching communication issues in cancer. In my first house job there were several occasions where I needed to break bad news and his techniques really worked. You could get past the diagnosis and discuss the real issues and the relief in patients and their families was palpable. The skills were probably the most useful that I learned at medical school at a time when there was much less emphasis on this in our training. I have subsequently attended courses to improve and develop communication skills and you are constantly learning with experience. At Wythenshawe there was a female consultant in medical oncology, Heather Anderson, who had, and still does, a uniquely holistic approach to her patients. I was inspired by her and have struggled to find similar role models subsequently. So, after enjoying general medicine and gaining membership I remained interested in oncology and got an SHO post at the Christie hospital. I have just spent 3 years as a research fellow and the pace of cancer research is staggering. I hope I will be part of an evolving speciality that sees dramatic advances in treatment by the time I retire. More parents are deciding against vaccination for their children and as a society we are increasingly sceptical about medical treatments. While it is good to have abandoned the blind faith in the medical establishment I think we have forgotten how serious many childhood diseases, TB, obstetric complications, etc. could be. I wonder whether people will ever forget how serious cancer could be?

I rate my greatest challenge and my best achievement so far, to be on the same career trajectory that I started on before having two children. Unfortunately I cannot say that my decision to have children and do a PhD was met with no prejudice. This was disappointing to encounter but not entirely unexpected. I think I might have changed track if my husband had not been a medic (Clinical Genetics) also doing a PhD. We met at the end of the 3rd year in Manchester and have always enjoyed a healthy degree of competition. We did membership (part 2) the same year we planned our wedding and friends were concerned that we wouldn't speak to each other and call off the wedding if one of us failed!! Our careers have now diverged however, Bill knows how much passion I have for oncology and this has encouraged me to maintain my chosen route although I'm still not quite sure whether I'll get to the destination I would like.

Having children has taught me a lot about the unpredictability that patients and their relatives often find so difficult to cope with. When I was pregnant for my first child I was doing a very busy job (there are now 8 Calman specialist registrars for that post!) I thrived on it but had been getting very tired. I phoned personnel to ask whether I could stop the on call rota after 28 weeks and continue working during the day to 36 weeks. I was told (by a mother) that previous doctors had managed on call to term. However, the following Monday I started to bleed after the morning ward round and a low lying placenta was diagnosed. I had to take sick leave for the remaining 3 months of the pregnancy and after sleeping continuously for the first 2 weeks, trundled into work until just before term to do desk work finishing some research projects. I was terribly frustrated and felt that I hadn't managed to 'do it all' and live up to the superwoman expectation – even though I attended an interview at the Cancer Research Campaign in London and was awarded a research fellowship when 35 weeks pregnant. A later scan showed that the placenta was in the right place and I think the bleeding was mainly due to overwork and exhaustion. It took me a long time to recover from that sense of failure. However, I was in a research post for my second pregnancy and from day one took regular breaks, ate frequently and rested well in the evenings. I worked till 39 weeks when my non-medical colleagues in the lab kicked me out with the fear that I might deliver in it (my first labour was 2 hours long). So, although pregnancy is not an illness, we should beware the anecdotes like 'Dr E was still performing emergency surgery at 38 weeks...' I recently heard of a house officer who requested to come off the cardiac arrest team when 34 weeks pregnant and was told she would not be signed up for full GMC registration if she did not remain on the team. I returned to work 10 weeks after delivery on both occasions and am currently on a (partly self-inflicted) 'family unfriendly' mission to complete my PhD and associated publications. I would advocate and encourage longer maternity leave or at least, reduced hours for 'early returners.'

My partner does a significant share of the childcare. He works in medical genetics led by Professor Donnai who is enlightened in encouraging a family friendly working practice, with some flexibility provided the work is done. My friends say I am very lucky because Bill does so much, but I know that if he had met someone who was willing to do it all for him he would have been equally happy to take a back seat in terms of domestic duties. You do have to be proactive in training your partner if you want to, or you need to be rich and employ some staff! (or be poor and employ some staff). The last thing the Health Service needs are frazzled doctors who haven't got their home lives sorted out.

I have often thought I should perhaps have a less busy job because then it definitely would be easier, but at the same time I thrive, definitely tick on having a busy schedule work-wise and I think that makes me probably better as a mother when I am at home. I'm constantly thinking about childcare arrangements, I'm not sure what the perfect arrangement is at all. I think female doctors with children need to continue discussing and supporting other doctors about the options. At one stage I thought nursery was best and nanny for the early months, but I'm really not sure now what is best at all. It's been really helpful speaking to the Medical Women's Federation doctors who have been through it and are now becoming grandmothers, because I think they globally pick up the feel that if you are just generally happy at home and do spend quality time regardless, and as long as your child-care is safe and not neglectful in any way and your children seem quite happy with it, then that's the best you can do and the rest is in the lap of the gods or whatever. Which is reassuring to know because I think we're in such a controlled society now and I think for thirty-something mothers across all careers, there's this real feeling having children is becoming very commercialised with all the stuff you can buy, baby accessories and so on, some very good, but some completely unnecessary. They definitely portray this, 'You can combine a career with a baby,' and the sort of perfect baby image, untired, unstressed mother with time for a facial once a week. There are huge pressures and you feel you should be able to control that and have perfect childcare and if you don't, then it's a disaster. It's quite difficult to fight against your sort of innate feeling that all these things aren't so important when you're being bombarded with messages. I think it is very difficult, like the breast versus bottle debate that becomes a huge issue and then I remember that myself and my husband were both bottle-fed from day one.

What advice would I offer to young people contemplating medicine as a career? It is a career with many pathways and opportunities that requires a high degree of motivation. You have to like people and an ability to enjoy working in a team is increasingly important. You no longer benefit so much if you can live on minimal sleep as working hours seem to be much improved in the early years post qualification but there are still problems with work intensity. I spent all my summers at University doing waitressing and bar jobs and this was the best preparation for house jobs since there is actually little difference in the organisational skills needed to wait on busy tables versus requests for venflons and blood tests! I don't think medicine is a particularly difficult subject and most courses are decreasing the volume of rote learning. It is a vocational course to be enjoyed and clinical training requires an open mind. Often there is no clear right and wrong in the management of patients, and the difficulty lies in balancing risks and benefits of treatment, and communicating that effectively to the patient. So medicine should be viewed as an art and not just a science. It is a very privileged and often humbling career that opens as many doors as you allow it to. On thinking about it I wouldn't like to go through medical school again, especially the anatomy. It seems completely absurd now to have been chopping up all those cadavers. I don't use any of that knowledge at all. But then I didn't become a surgeon after all.

DR. ROWAN KERR-LIDDELL
Paediatric Senior House Officer

Rowan is our youngest member, born in 1974. She qualified in 1999 after studying at St. Andrews and Manchester. There are no other doctors in her family. She went to a state school in Bakewell, Derbyshire, where her ambition to read medicine was not well received. It was predicted that she would be unable to obtain the necessary grades, but, presented with this challenge, she was delighted to demonstrate her true capabilities.

She accepted a place at St Andrews without ever having seen it. After some misgivings on discovering its location she quickly settled in and was extremely happy there. She also enjoyed the clinical training in Manchester, especially the paediatrics in which she intends to make her career. She has obtained some careers guidance in conversation with paediatricians but not from formal careers advisers.

Her pre-registration surgical job was split between urology at Withington and colorectal surgery at Wythenshawe, then she did general medicine at Royal Bolton Hospital. She has now begun paediatrics with a year at Wythenshawe prior to a two-year rotation at the Manchester Children's Hospitals. She has no complaints about working conditions and considers the rotas fair and reasonable. When asked to do extra on-call recently she was offered extra holiday in lieu, which she found perfectly satisfactory. She has not encountered any discrimination against women.

Rowan hopes to settle down and have a family in due course and is aware that this can be difficult to fit in with medicine – one reason why she joined MWF, to turn to when she feels the need. She intends to complete her higher training full-time if possible, but knows about flexible training and will investigate if the need arises.

In the meantime she plans to tackle the Membership and keep up her hobbies of rock-climbing, cycling and socialising with friends.

DR. SARAH WHITEHEAD
Medical Senior House Officer

Sarah was a mature student at Manchester and qualified in 1999. This medical school was not her first choice but she has no regrets about coming here. There are other doctors in her family and she was not discouraged from trying for medicine either at home or at her state school.

She hopes eventually to make a career in microbiology and plans to continue working full-time; 'settling down' and having children are not necessarily on her agenda. She is aware of the flexible training scheme and has had the benefit of careers advice, but cannot ignore her own observations. She writes:

'I think it is still much easier for a female doctor to further her career if she remains childless and that the same does not apply to male doctors. I would like to see career breaks and part-time work completely accepted for both sexes without any stigma attached.'

Sarah did a pre-registration orthopaedic house-job at Trafford General Hospital and then moved on to a medical job at Withington. She finds the rotas and working conditions satisfactory on the whole but would like to see the system changed:

'I feel it would be quite reasonable (as in Australia) for us to work a 40-hour week for the current salary. This would involve training and employing more doctors and, if necessary, raising income tax to pay for it.'

Though very short of free time at the moment Sarah relaxes when she can by reading, travelling and eating out. She appreciates the influence of the Medical Women's Federation:

'I have met many charming and interesting lady doctors who have made me realise how much progress has been made for women in medicine by such groups. I haven't experienced any sexism, but I am very junior. It occurs at consultant level in some specialities; women doctors can contribute by getting to the top and changing things. So they can press for family friendly careers and have more to gain from this than many male doctors.'

Sarah is currently using her computer skills to develop a website for the Federation.

She feels that the NHS is very understaffed at present and therefore unable to provide an optimum service. She considers the greatest challenges to medicine in the future include finding cures or effective treatments for arthritis, heart disease and cancer, but also:

'In this country, at least, finding a way to stop acute hospital beds being occupied by people who should be in community rest or nursing homes. I took very little interest in politics before I started work as an NHS doctor, but I now recognise that only political will can resolve the problems of understaffing and inappropriate use of acute resources. Also the ethical use of genetic techniques and IVF – an issue for society as a whole, not just doctors.'

Sarah strongly encourages anyone with a real ambition to read medicine to persevere with their applications to medical school.

'There is such a wide variety of jobs after qualification that there should be something to suit all types of people. If you don't get an offer from a medical school, get the best possible A-level results, do hospital work to show you are committed and reapply next year. And don't forget the Irish universities – you can apply to all of them and one of them made me a firm offer when my A-level results were published.'

CONCLUSIONS

It has been a privilege to bring together the foregoing stories. All are unique but reflect, to some extent, prevailing attitudes and circumstances as they have changed down the years. At the instigation of colleagues I will illustrate this further by comparing my own history as a GP with that of my daughter Sophie who is a paediatric specialist registrar. We qualified in 1964 and 1991 respectively.

I came from a non-medical family. My parents were enthusiastic about my decision to read medicine but knew very little about the realities of that choice. With doctors as parents, on the other hand, Sophie had a good idea what she was letting herself in for, but this obviously did not deter her. In fact I believe she benefited from the kind of insight that I had conspicuously lacked when it came to planning a career, and learnt from my mistakes. Although I wanted to be a doctor I had only the haziest notions about the different specialties and the only female doctors I had come across were GPs. One of them probably saved my life with M&B when I had pneumonia at the age of three.

I attended Accrington High School for Girls and achieved good enough A-levels to obtain a state scholarship, but was too young to go to university straightaway. Because I had a burning desire to go to Oxford I stayed on at school to take the entrance exam. It was one of the best moments of my life when I heard I had got in. In her turn, sitting the entrance exam even before she had taken A-levels, Sophie obtained a scholarship to Oxford from Cheadle Hulme High School, a mixed comprehensive. So state schools did not prevent either of us from realising our aspirations but in both cases were actively helpful in preparing us for the exams.

I had a wonderful time at Oxford doing preclinical studies and a degree in animal physiology. Our teachers included Hans Krebs, famous for his cycle, and Howard Florey who developed penicillin. Then I did my clinical training at St Thomas's in London, whereas Sophie stayed on in Oxford. St Thomas's in the early 60's was hardly a female-friendly medical school but I enjoyed my time there and the excitement of living in London. Careers advice was totally lacking. None of the very few women in my year got house-jobs in Thomas's, because a woman house officer in the previous year had become pregnant in the middle of her job, shock, horror! However I am glad to say she later became a consultant at St Thomas's.

I found pre-registration jobs in London peripheral hospitals and then took a post as SHO in clinical pathology at St George's, because I had liked pathology as a student and won a prize for it. Unfortunately the job offered little or no training. I spent all my days cross-matching blood and nights on call trying to do emergency investigations on antiquated equipment, because residents were not let loose on the fancy new auto-analysers. The beautiful old hospital at Hyde Park Corner soon began to feel like a prison and my ambition withered and died. By this time I had encountered a few female consultants but all seemed to be terribly dedicated, single and childless.

Feeling disillusioned with medicine, I decided I would prefer to have children. I had met my future husband in the first year at Oxford and we got married a year before finals. He did well at Guy's and was set on a career in paediatrics. And so I happily abandoned medicine and worked at home for the next three years, as a maths tutor for Gabbitas-Thring and then as a copywriter for Roche, while our two daughters came along. I then accepted an offer of a part-time GP partnership, starting when my second baby was not quite six weeks old. Alternate weekends on call were fairly taxing and I was glad of my husband's assistance. On one occasion he did a home visit for me and discovered a case of meningococcal meningitis. Although I had never intended to go into general practice I took to it quite well and was fortunate to land on my feet in this way, without training and with little relevant experience. I had to learn on the job which was still the norm at that time when the first vocational training courses were only just beginning. Nowadays it is not possible to drop into general practice without all the appropriate training although one can still be a GP principal at a younger age than one can be a hospital consultant. With hindsight I regret not attempting the MRCP as this would have given me a wider choice of possible careers.

Sophie had the time of her life as a student and still managed to get a first class degree. Unlike myself, she had definite career plans and stuck to them. She decided to specialise in paediatrics and set about passing membership as soon as possible after qualifying, obtaining good training posts and working extremely hard. She did not embark on motherhood for a few years so could continue working full-time. Since starting a family she has completed a DPhil and has been able to switch to flexible training without any difficulty. In due course she may seek a part-time or jobsharing consultant post.

A recent report from the three Royal Colleges of Physicians recommended that there should be "a huge expansion in opportunities for consultants to work part-time or to jobshare, far more out-of-hours hospital crèches, and an end to the assumption that a medical career requires commitment at the expense of family life. Women are being held back in the race to become senior hospital doctors because of the 'working all hours' culture that remains in the NHS." Professor Carol Black who chaired the report also said, "The working lives of doctors.. will not improve without a substantial increase in the total workforce." Exactly what many of us have been saying for years!

Fitting in work with children was never easy. A fact of life which working mothers need to grasp is that you cannot do everything yourself. In the the 60's and 70's we all thought we should, thanks to people like Shirley Conran who wrote the book entitled "Superwoman." On the contrary, you should harness all the help you can get, starting with your husband. When I was growing up most husbands felt it reflected badly on themselves if their wives went out to work, and expected them to shoulder the whole of the domestic burden. My own mother never worked after I was born and would have liked to find a job during the 1950's, but was strongly discouraged by my father. My husband has not exactly played a major domestic role but has always been very supportive. Sophie is married to a research neuroscientist whose hours are flexible and he takes an active part in looking after their offspring and domestic responsibilities generally – a New Man. Our other daughter, Anna, is a full-time hospital dentist in Pittsburgh and has two children. Her husband is a medical resident and is also a New Man when he can stay awake. This is not the place for their story but I can say that hours and rotas in US hospitals are considerably worse than ours and maternity leave is almost non-existent.

Childcare has always been a crucial issue for working mothers. In my time such authorities as John Bowlby were maintaining that infants suffer psychological damage if looked after by anyone other than their mothers. This made it very hard for young mothers to feel happy about going back to work. Nowadays such attitudes are not so prevalent and most people believe children get on perfectly well in the care of others as long as they are competent. A grandma can be an ideal carer, if available. Anna is fortunate enough to have a willing mother-in-law. Other family members can also be a help, even if only as a backstop for emergencies. My own childminder was just a local lady with children of her own but no qualifications; Sophie, perhaps more wisely, shares a trained daily nanny with another family. Others will prefer a nursery. The important thing is to be sure that you feel comfortable with the care you have chosen. A recent survey showed that the mother's morale is the most important factor affecting her child's wellbeing whether she is working or not. It seems outrageous that there is still no tax allowance for the cost of childcare.

The income of newly qualified NHS doctors is modest compared with some other jobs, but better than it used to be. My first job was paid at the rate of £600 a year – a paltry sum even in 1965. At least nowadays a junior doctor can afford to pay for childcare and cleaning. These expenses should be regarded as an investment for the future: money worth spending to maintain quality home life while securing a worthwhile career – maybe a large part of your income at this stage but you should be able to make up for it later. And be sure to have good holidays to re-charge your batteries.

Career progress has to fit in with your partner, if you have one, or vice versa. I had to leave my GP post in South London when my husband became a consultant in Manchester. Once here, I had a series of locums and assistant posts and was a partner for a time in an unsatisfactory practice which I was glad to leave. To extend my skills I took courses in family planning and hypnosis. I also made use of the Doctors' Retainer Scheme. Through this I was introduced to a reputable training practice in which I eventually became a partner and was happy to remain for the rest of my career.

Unlike some of my colleagues I was also more than happy to retire. Although I derived a lot of satisfaction from my work I decided I had had enough, at the time when fundamental changes were being forced on general practice. I was particularly averse to the decision of my partners to go into fundholding. (I am glad that the system has now changed again). It is a joy to have more time to devote to both family and outside interests. At last I have made myself conversant with computers and even go to a gym. I enjoy seeing my grandchildren and helping to run two local choirs. Also I have always been keen on travelling and hope to explore new horizons in years to come.

My advice to those considering medicine as a career: you need compassion and the capacity for hard work and handling responsibility. You should expect to be frequently exhausted, worried and distressed. At the same time your work would be enormously satisfying and always worthwhile. As our accounts show, women doctors' prospects in every field are improving all the time though in some areas there is still a long way to go. Discrimination has markedly lessened and part-timers have a much fairer deal, sometimes even to the chagrin of their full-time colleagues. There is perhaps a better chance than ever before of combining a fulfilling career in medicine with a normal family life, if that is your choice.

Dr Mary Hambleton (Editor)

APPENDIX (1)
The Questionnaire – Manchester MWF Millennium Project

Here are a few questions to give an outline of your medical career.

Do not feel obliged to answer all of the questions.

Please put a tick against topics you would be willing to say more about.

Your name ....

(If you would prefer your name not to be quoted please tick here ....)

When and where did you qualify?

Was this medical school your first choice?

Have you since wished you had been at a different one?

Was it your own decision to study medicine?

Were there other doctors in your family?

Did you experience any discouragement about applying for medicine – at home or at school?

Was your school in the state system or private?

After qualifying, did you have any difficulties in obtaining posts?

Which field of medicine have you mainly worked in?

Did your eventual career path result from long-held preference or seizing opportunity?

Did you change your mind many times along the way?

What are your principal outside interests?

If you have married, how long before or after qualifying?

If you have a husband or partner, is he a doctor too?

If you have children, how long before or after qualifying did the first arrive?

Was this as planned? (You do not have to answer this question!)

With hindsight, would you have changed the timing of your family?

How much time did you take off work after giving birth?

Has coping with home and children been difficult to fit in with work?

Have you had to pay for childcare or relied on family or friends?

Have any of your children followed you into Medicine?

What is the greatest professional challenge you have had to meet?

What professional achievement has pleased you the most?

What was your greatest disappointment in your career?

How do you rate the NHS?

If you can remember healthcare before the NHS please compare.

What do you regard as the greatest challenges for medicine in the future?

How do you rate the contribution women doctors can make?

How have you been influenced by belonging to MWF?

What advice would you offer to young people contemplating medicine as a career?

APPENDIX (2)
Abbreviations

A&E	Accident and Emergency
AGM	Annual General Meeting
BA	Bachelor of Arts
BCG	Bacille Calmette-Guérin (vaccine for tuberculosis)
BPhil	Bachelor of Philosophy
BSc	Bachelor of Science
ChM	Master of Surgery
CSF	Cerebrospinal fluid
CV	Curriculum vitae (history of training and career)
D&V	Diarrhoea and vomiting
DMRD	Diploma in Medical Radio-Diagnosis
DM	Doctor of Medicine
DPhil	Doctor of Philosophy
DPH	Diploma in Public Health
ENT	Ear, Nose and Throat
FHSA	Family Health Services Authority
FP	Family Planning
FPC	Family Practitioner Committee
FRCGP	Fellow of the Royal College of General Practitioners
FRCS	Fellow of the Royal College of Surgeons
FRCSE	Fellow of the Royal College of Surgeons of Edinburgh
GMC	General Medical Council
IT	Information Technology
LMC	Local Medical Committee
LRAM	Licentiate of the Royal Academy of Music
M&B	Sulphapyridine, early antibacterial drug made by May & Baker
MB	Bachelor of Medicine
MBE	Member of the Order of the British Empire
MRCGP	Member of the Royal College of General Practitioners
MRCPath	Member of the Royal College of Pathologists
MRCP	Member of the Royal College of Physicians
MRI	Manchester Royal Infirmary
MSc	Master of Science
MSD	Merck, Sharp & Dohme
MSF	Medicin sans Frontières (medicine without frontiers)

MWF	Medical Women's Federation
NHS	National Health Service
OBE	Officer of the Order of the British Empire
PCG	Primary Care Group
PhD	Doctor of Philosophy
PLAB	Professional & Linguistic Assessment Board
RCO	Resident Clinical Officer
SHO	Senior House Officer
SR	Senior Registrar
SpR	Specialist Registrar
UCCA	Universities Central Council on Admissions
VSO	Voluntary Service Overseas